# AMBULATORY PATIENT CARE

By

LINDA B. CHITWOOD RN, CRNA, MS

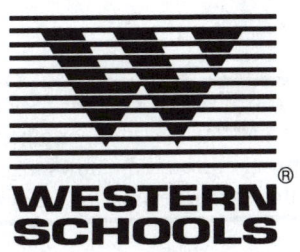

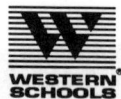

21 Bristol Drive
South Easton, MA 02375
1-800-618-1670

**ABOUT THE AUTHOR.**

Linda B. Chitwood, RN, CRNA, MS is a nurse anesthetist and medical writer in Memphis, Tennessee. The author of a number of articles in the health care specialties, she has published articles in *Nursing, Journal of Clinical Psychiatry and Health Care News,* as well as consumer publications. She is also the author of other continuing education courses for Western Schools.

**ABOUT THE SUBJECT MATTER EXPERT:**

Lillian C. Cotterman, RN, BSN is currently clinical coordinator of Same-Day-Surgery of Outpatient Services at St. Francis Hospital, Memphis, Tennessee. She has 26 years experience working as an operating room, intensive-care post-surgery, post-anesthesia care unit, and ambulatory care nurse.

**Copy Editor:** Janet Rushford, RN, MA
**Graphic Artist:** Kathy Johnson
**Typesetter:** Gwen Nichols
**Indexed:** Sylvia Coates

WESTERN SCHOOLS' courses are designed to provide nursing professionals with general information to assist in their practices and professional development. The information provided in these courses and course books is based on research and consultation with nursing and medical authorities, and is, to the best of WESTERN SCHOOLS' knowledge, current and accurate. However, the courses and course books are offered with the understanding that WESTERN SCHOOLS is not engaged in rendering legal, nursing, medical or other professional advice. WESTERN SCHOOLS' courses and course books are not a substitute for seeking professionadvise or conducting individual research. In applying the information provided in the courses and course books to individual circumstances, all recommendations must be considered in light of the unique circumstances of each situation. The course books are intended solely for your use, and not for the benefit of providing advice or recommendations to third parties. WESTERN SCHOOLS disclaims my responsibility for any adverse consequences resulting from the failure to seek nursing, medical or other professional advice, or to conduct independent research. WESTERN SCHOOLS further disclaims my responsibility for updating or revising any programs or publications presented, published, distributed or sponsored by WESTERN SCHOOLS unless otherwise agreed to as part of an individual purchase contract.

**ISBN-**1-878025-63-5
**Library of Congress Catalog Card Number -** 94-60526

COPYRIGHT© 1994 - WESTERN SCHOOLS, INC. ALL RIGHTS RESERVED. No part of this material may be reprinted, reproduced, transmitted, stored in a retrieval system, or otherwise utilized, in any form or by any means electronic or mechanical, including photocopying or recording, now existing or hereinafter invented, nor may any part of this course be used for teaching without the written permission from the publisher and the author.

# IMPORTANT: Read these instructions *BEFORE* proceeding!

Enclosed with your course book you will find the FasTrax™ answer sheet. Use this form to answer all the final exam questions that appear in this course book. If you are completing more than one course, be sure to write your answers on the appropriate answer sheet. Full instructions and complete grading details are printed on the FasTrax instruction sheet, also enclosed with your order. Please review them before starting. *If you are mailing your answer sheet(s) to Western Schools, we recommend you make a copy as a backup.*

## ABOUT THIS COURSE

A "Pretest" is provided with each course to test your current knowledge base regarding the subject matter contained within this course. Your "Final Exam" is a multiple choice examination. **You will find the exam questions at the end of each chapter.** Some smaller hour courses include the exam at the end of the book.

In the event the course has less than 100 questions, mark your answers to the questions in the course book and leave the remaining answer boxes on the FasTrax answer sheet blank. **Use a black pen to fill in your answer sheet.**

## A PASSING SCORE

You must score 70% or better in order to pass this course and receive your Certificate of Completion. Should you fail to achieve the required score, we will send you an additional FasTrax answer sheet so that you may make a second attempt to pass the course. Western Schools will allow you three chances to pass the same course...*at no extra charge!* After three failed attempts to pass the same course, your file will be closed.

## RECORDING YOUR HOURS

Please monitor the time it takes to complete this course using the handy log sheet on the other side of this page. See below for transferring study hours to the course evaluation.

## COURSE EVALUATIONS

In this course book you will find a short evaluation about the course you are soon to complete. This information is vital to providing the school with feedback on this course. The course evaluation answer section is in the lower right hand corner of the FasTrax answer sheet marked "Evaluation" with answers marked 1–25. Your answers are important to us, please take five minutes to complete the evaluation.

On the back of the FasTrax instruction sheet there is additional space to make any comments about the course, the school, and suggested new curriculum. Please mail the FasTrax instruction sheet, with your comments, back to Western Schools in the envelope provided with your course order.

## TRANSFERRING STUDY TIME

Upon completion of the course, transfer the total study time from your log sheet to question #25 in the Course Evaluation. The answers will be in ranges, please choose the proper hour range that best represents your study time. You MUST log your study time under question #25 on the course evaluation.

## EXTENSIONS

You have 2 years from the date of enrollment to complete this course. A six (6) month extension may be purchased. If after 30 months from the original enrollment date you do not complete the course, *your file will be closed and no certificate can be issued.*

## CHANGE OF ADDRESS?

In the event you have moved during the completion of this course please call our student services department at 1-800-618-1670 and we will update your file.

## A GUARANTEE YOU'LL GIVE HIGH HONORS TO

If any continuing education course fails to meet your expectations or if you are not satisfied in any manner, for any reason, you may return it for an exchange or a refund (less shipping and handling) within 30 days. Software, video and audio courses must be returned unopened.

*Thank you for enrolling at Western Schools!*

WESTERN SCHOOLS
P.O. Box 1930
Brockton, MA 02303
(800) 618-1670

# AMBULATORY PATIENT CARE

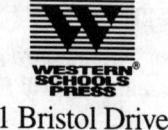

21 Bristol Drive
South Easton, MA 02375

Please use this log to total the number of hours you spend reading the text and taking the final examination (use 50-min hours).

| Date | Hours Spent |
|---|---|
| 1/11 | / |
| | |

**TOTAL** [ ]

**Please log your study hours with submission of your final exam.** To log your study time, fill in the appropriate circle under question 25 of the FasTrax® answer sheet under the "Evaluation" section.

**PLEASE LOG YOUR STUDY HOURS WITH SUBMISSION OF YOUR FINAL EXAM.** Please choose which best represents the total study hours it took to complete this 30 hour course.

  A. less than 25 hours
  B. 25–28 hours
  C. 29–32 hours
  D. greater than 32 hours

# AMBULATORY PATIENT CARE

## WESTERN SCHOOLS' NURSING
## CONTINUING EDUCATION EVALUATION

Instructions: Mark your answers to the following questions with a black pen on the "Evaluation" section of your FasTrax® answer sheet provided with this course. You should not return this sheet. Please use the scale below to rate the following statements:

- **A** Agree Strongly
- **B** Agree Somewhat
- **C** Disagree Somewhat
- **D** Disagree Strongly

The course content met the following education objectives:

1. *[A]* Addressed the changes in the delivery of health care that have occurred in this century, and how those changes have led to increased utilization of ambulatory care and what to expect in future trends in ambulatory patient care.

2. *[A]* Distinguished between the different types of facilities where ambulatory patient care is provided, described the relative advantages and disadvantages of each, and recognized how the different types of facilities may influence nursing practice.

3. *[A]* Recognized the steps of the nursing process and identified how that process may be shaped by the special needs of the ambulatory patient.

4. *[B]* Explained how to discern which patients and procedures are ideally suited to ambulatory care, which are more appropriately treated in an inpatient setting, and how that decision is influenced.

5. *[A]* Defined general anesthesia, recognized fundamental aspects of the administration of general anesthesia, specified the pharmacologic agents commonly used in the ambulatory setting, and then based on this knowledge, explained how to plan nursing care for the ambulatory patient undergoing general anesthesia.

6. *[A]* Defined regional and local anesthesia and conscious sedation, recognized the pharmacologic agents commonly used in these anesthetics, and explained how to plan nursing care for the ambulatory patient undergoing one of these anesthetics.

*[A]* 7. Explained how to plan nursing care for the patient preparing to undergo an ambulatory procedure.

*[A]* 8. Prepared you to implement nursing care for the patient during an ambulatory care procedure.

9. *[A]* Explained how to care for a patient during the period of time immediately following an ambulatory care procedure.

*[A]* 10. Explained discharge procedures for the ambulatory patient.

11. Described how to differentiate among and deliver care to ambulatory patients who have special needs.

12. Described the implementation process for ambulatory patients undergoing different types of surgery.

A 13. Explained how to plan and implement nursing care for ambulatory patients undergoing common diagnostic and therapeutic procedures.

A 14. The content of this course was relevant to the objectives.

A 15. This offering met my professional education needs.

A 16. The information in this offering is relevant to my professional work setting.

A 17. The course was generally well written and the subject matter explained thoroughly? (If no please explain on the back of the FasTrax instruction sheet.)

A 18. The content of this course was appropriate for home study.

A 19. The final examination was well written and at an appropriate level for the content of the course.

Please complete the following research questions in order to help us better meet your educational needs. Pick the ONE answer which is most appropriate.

20. What nursing shift do you most commonly work?
    - A. (circled) Morning Shift (Any shift starting after 3:00am or before 11:00am)
    - B. Day/Afternoon Shift (Any shift starting after 11:00am or before 7:00pm)
    - C. Night Shift (Any shift starting after 7:00pm or before 3:00am)
    - D. I work rotating shifts

21. What was the SINGLE most important reason you chose this course?
    - A. Low Price
    - B. New or Newly revised course
    - C. (circled) High interest/Required course topic
    - D. Number of Contact Hours Needed

22. Where do you work? (If your place of employment is not listed below, please leave this question blank.)
    - A. (circled) Hospital
    - B. Medical Clinic/Group Practice/HMO/Office setting
    - C. Long Term Care/Rehabilitation Facility/Nursing Home
    - D. Home Health Care Agency

23. Which field do you specialize in?
    - A. (circled) Medical/Surgical
    - B. Geriatrics
    - C. Pediatrics/Neonatal
    - D. Other

24. For your last renewal, how many months BEFORE your license expiration date did you order your course materials?
    - A. (circled) 1–3 months
    - B. 4–6 months
    - C. 7–12 months
    - D. Greater than 12 months

25. **PLEASE LOG YOUR STUDY HOURS WITH SUBMISSION OF YOUR FINAL EXAM.** Please choose which best represents the total study hours it took to complete this 30 hour course.
    - A. (circled) less than 25 hours
    - B. 25–28 hours
    - C. 29–32 hours
    - D. greater than 32 hours

# CONTENTS

**Pretest vxi**
**Introduction xv**

### Chapter 1  The Revolution in Ambulatory Patient Care 1
Introduction 1
The Development of Ambulatory Services 2
Ambulatory Care: Advantages and Disadvantages 3
Advantages 3
Disadvantages 4
Alternatives to Ambulatory Care 4
The Future of Ambulatory Care 5
Summary 5
Critical Concepts 6
Exam Questions 7

### Chapter 2  The Ambulatory Facility 9
Introduction 9
Types of Ambulatory Patient Care Facilities 9
Hospitals 10
Freestanding Units 11
Physicians Offices 11
Standards for Ambulatory Patient Care Facilities 12
The Ambulatory Care Facility 12
The Environment 12
Disaster Preparation 13
Security 13
Summary 13
Critical Concepts 14
Exam Questions 15

### Chapter 3  The Nursing Process and the Ambulatory Patient 17
Introduction 17
Ambulatory Care and the Nursing Process 18
Assessment 18
Diagnosis 18
Planning 19
Implementation 19
Evaluation 19
Special Considerations in Planning Care for the Ambulatory Patient 20
Standards of Care 21
Legal Considerations 21
Advanced Directive 21

Patients' Rights and Responsibility 21
Summary 21
Critical Concepts 21
Exam Questions 23

## Chapter 4    Selection of the Ambulatory Patient 25
Introduction 25
Selecting Patients for Ambulatory Care 25
Age 26
Health Status 26
Nature of the Procedure 27
Support System 28
Third-Party Payer 28
Physicians 28
Nursing Considerations 28
Summary 29
Critical Concepts 29
Exam Questions 30

## Chapter 5    Considerations in Ambulatory Anesthesia: General Anesthesia 31
Introduction 31
General Anesthesia 32
Induction 32
Maintenance 33
Emergence 33
Special Considerations 33
Indications 34
Contraindications 34
Intravenous Agents Used During Anesthesia 35
Narcotics 35
Tranquilizers 37
Agonist-antagonist Agents 37
Non-narcotic,Non-barbiturate Hypnotic Agents 38
Barbiturates 38
Dissociative Agent 38
Neuromuscular Blocking Agents 39
Inhalation Agents Used In General Anesthesia 40
Inhalation Anesthetic Agents 40
Carrier Gases 41
Monitoring in Anesthesia 41
Nursing Strategies for the Ambulatory Patient Undergoing General Anesthesia 42
Summary 45
Critical Concepts 45
Exam Questions 47

# CONTENTS - AMBULATORY PATIENT CARE

## Chapter 6 Considerations in Ambulatory Anesthesia: Regional Anesthesia, Local Anesthesia & Sedation 49

Introduction 49
Regional Anesthesia 50
Indications 50
Contraindications 50
Regional Anesthesia Techniques 51
Spinal Anesthesia 51
Epidural Anesthesia and Analgesia 52
Intravenous Regional Anesthesia 53
Nerve Blocks 53
Local Anesthesia 54
Monitored Anesthesia Care (MAC) & Conscious Sedation 55
Pharmacologic Agents 56
Nursing Strategies 56
Summary 59
Critical Concepts 59
Study Questions 60

## Chapter 7 Preparing the Patient for the Procedure 61

Introduction 61
Patient Preparation in the Ambulatory Setting 62
The Perioperative Team 62
Nurses 62
Physicians 62
Anesthesia Team 62
Ancillary Personnel 63
Patient Preparation: Assessment and Planning 63
Reason for Admission 64
Review of Body Systems and Current Health Status 64
List of All Medications 64
Allergies 65
Social History 65
Emotional Status 65
Prosthetics 65
Time of Last Oral Intake 65
Height and Weight 65
Physical Exam 65
Baseline Vital Signs 68
Planning 68
Preoperative and Preprocedure Teaching 68
Teaching and Learning 69
Content 69
Documentation 69
Preanesthesia Evaluation 69
Preanesthesia Interview 70

Physical Examination 71
Anesthesia Care Plan 71
Preanesthesia Medication 71
Tranquilizers 72
Aspiration Prophylaxis 73
Narcotics 73
Antiemetics 73
Anticholinergics 73
Antibiotics 73
Nursing Strategies 73
Summary 76
Critical Concepts 76
Exam Questions 77

### Chapter 8   Nursing Care of the Patient During the Procedure 79
Introduction 79
Preparing the Environment 79
The Procedure Suite 80
Ambience 81
Caring for the Patient 81
Admission 81
Assessment 81
Positioning 81
Monitoring 82
Preparing the Site 82
Documentation 82
Family and Support Persons Care 82
Discharge From the Procedure Room 85
Nursing Strategies 85
Summary 89
Critical Concepts 89
Exam Questions 91

### Chapter 9   Nursing Care of the Patient Afterf the Procedure 93
Introduction 93
Recovery from Anesthesia 93
General Anesthesia 94
Regional Anesthesia 94
Local Anesthesia 95
After the Procedure 95
Admission to the PACU 97
Complications 97
Documentation 99
Family and Support Persons Care 99
Discharge from the Postanesthesia Room 99

# CONTENTS - AMBULATORY PATIENT CARE

Nursing Strategies 101
Summary 104
Critical Concepts 104
Exam Questions 105

## Chapter 10  Discharging The Patient 107
Introduction 107
Recovery Phase 2 107
Nursing Assessment 108
Common Complications 108
Discharge 110
Follow-up Care 112
Nursing Strategies 112
Summary 115
Critical Concepts 115
Exam Questions 116

## Chapter 11  Special Ambulatory Patients 117
Introduction 117
Ambutatory Pediatric Patients 118
Preparation 118
During the Procedure 119
Aftercare 119
Ambulatory Geriatric Patients 120
Preparation 122
During the Procedure 122
Aftercare 122
Other Patients With Special Needs 122
Impaired Patients 122
Trauma and Emergency Patients 123
Nursing Strategies 123
Summary 126
Critical Concepts 126
Exam Questions 127

## Chapter 12  Ambulatory Nursing Considerations in the Surgical Specialties 129
Introduction 129
Ambulatory Surgery 130
Gynecology & Obstetrics 130
Intra-abdominal Surgery 131
Intra-uterine Procedures 131
Cervical and Vaginal Procedures 132
Genitalia 132
Nursing Strategies 32
Orthopedics& Podiatry 134

Arthroscopic Procedures 135
Nursing Strategies 135
Plastic Surgery 137
Reconstruction, Revision, Excision and Aesthetic Procedures 137
Nursing Strategies 138
Otolaryngology & Oral Surgery 138
Ear Procedures 139
Nose and Sinus Procedures 140
Throat Procedures 140
Oral Surgery 141
Nursing Strategies 141
Urology 143
General Urologic Procedures 143
Lithotripsy 143
Nursing Strategies 143
Ophthalmology 145
Extraocular Procedures 145
Intraocular Procedures 145
Nursing Strategies 145
Cardiovascular 147
General Surgery 147
Summary 147
Critical Concepts 147
Exam Questions 148

## Chapter 13   Nursing Considerations in Diagnostic and Therapeutic Procedures 151
Introduction 151
Diagnostic and Therapeutic Procedures 152
Gastrointestinal Procedures 152
Diagnostic Procedures 152
Therapeutic Procedures 153
Nursing Considerations 154
Radiologic Procedures 154
Diagnostic Procedures 156
Therapeutic Procedures 156
Nursing Strategies 156
Cardiac Procedures 157
Diagnostic Procedures 157
Therapeutic Procedures 158
Nursing Considerations 159
Obstetrical Procedures 159
Invasive Procedures 159
Non-invasive Procedures 160
Nursing Strategies 160
Parenteral Therapy 161

Chemotherapy 161
Nursing Strategies 161
Other Ambulatory Procedures 163
Pain Management 163
Nerve Blocks 163
Pulmonary Procedures 164
Summary 164
Critical Concepts 164
Exam Questions 165

**Chapter 14   Surgical and Anesthetic Emergencies 167**
Introduction 167
Surgical Emergencies 168
Anesthetic Emergencies 168
Airway Compromise 168
Cardiovascular Compromise 170
Nursing Strategies 171
Summary 174
Critical Concepts 175
Exam Questions 176

**Appendix A: Resources 177**

**Appendix B: Association of Operating Room Nurses Recommended Practices 179**

**Appendix C: Difficult Airway Algorithm 189**

**Bibliography 181**

**Suggested Reading List 193**

**Glossary 195**

**Index**

**Pretest Answer Key**

# PRETEST

Begin by taking the pretest. Compare your answers on the pretest to the answer key (located in the back of the book). Circle those test items that you missed. The pretest answer key indicates the course chapters where the content of that question is discussed.

Next, read each chapter. Focus special attention on the chapters where you made incorrect answer choices. Study questions are provided at the end of each chapter so you can assess your progress and understanding of the material.

1. A future trend in ambulatory care may include:

    a. Accepting sicker patients for ambulatory procedures
    b. Strictly limiting ambulatory services to healthy patients
    c. Asking patients provide their own meals and medications
    d. Denial of care to patients who do not comply with instructions

2. A key issue in determining where ambulatory care will be delivered is:

    a. Location
    b. Reputation
    c. Reimbursement
    d. Preference

3. Federal law requires that Medicare and Medicaid patients be informed of their right to make basic decisions about their health care. This is called:

    a. Classified Reimbursement
    b. Advance Directive
    c. Rationed Care
    d. Due Process

4. Your patient drives himself to the ambulatory surgery facility for knee surgery. He has made no plans to have a support person drive him home or care for him that night. The nurse should:

    a. Cancel the procedure
    b. Notify his physician
    c. Confiscate his car keys
    d. Call his mother

5. Which of these monitors assesses the amount of oxygen being delivered to the patient's lungs?

    a. Electrocardiogram
    b. Nerve stimulator
    c. Precordial stethoscope
    d. Inspired oxygen

6. In general, with modern anesthetic agents developed in the past few years, postoperative patients can expect to have:

    a. More pain
    b. Less pain
    c. More N & V
    d. Less N & V

7. Adults generally undergo which type of anesthesia induction?

   a. Intravenous
   b. Inhalation
   c. Mask
   d. Ether

8. Which of the following regional anesthetic techniques would be indicated for surgery on the hand?

   a. Subarachnoid block
   b. Epidural analgesia
   c. Bier block
   d. Caudal block

9. A local anesthetic used in epidural analgesia and anesthesia is

   a. Bupivicaine
   b. Cocaine
   c. Etomacaine
   d. Prilocaine

10. Which one of the following classes of drugs are strongly suspected to be teratogenic (cause malformations in the fetus)?

    a. Opioids
    b. Barbiturates
    c. enzodiazepines
    d. Hypnotics.

11. What is the weight of a 170-pound man in kilograms?

    a. 77
    b. 53
    c. 110
    d. 89

12. Which of the following lab reports would most likely result in cancellation of surgery?

    a. Potassium 2.6
    b. Hematocrit 33
    c. Platelet count 250,000.
    d. Urine pH 6

13. Which of the following will not help maintain asepsis in the Operating Room (OR)?

    a. Propping the door open
    b. Sterilizing equipment
    c. Prepping the operative site
    d. Using sterile technique

14. The final phase of general anesthesia is:

    a. Induction
    b. Maintenance
    c. Emergence
    d. Delirium

15. Postoperative patients seldom need to come to the PACU if they received only:

    a. Local anesthesia
    b. Conscious sedation
    c. Epidural anesthesia
    d. General anesthesia

16. Hypotension can cause which of the following in the postoperative patient?

    a. Pain
    b. Nausea
    c. Dsypnea
    d. Headache

17. Which of the following is often used to assess the patient's readiness for discharge?

    a. Breathalyzer tests
    b. Scoring criteria
    c. Hematocrit
    d. Financial analysis

18. The second most common cause of injury in the elderly is:

    a. Falls
    b. Motor vehicle accidents
    c. Heart disease
    d. Burns

19. You are caring for a 62-year-old ambulatory postop cataract extraction patient. When her husband arrives to pick her up, he is clearly intoxicated. You should:

    a. Take your patient to his car
    b. Call the patient's neighbor
    c. Notify his employer and have him arrested
    d. Refuse to release your patient to his care

20. During your follow-up call the day after surgery, a patient who had a laparoscopy complains that her shoulder hurts. You tell her to call her doctor if this pain doesn't resolve in a day or two, because this is:

    a. Common after laparoscopy
    b. A serious complication
    c. Unusual after laparoscopy
    d. Due to a pneumothorax

21. Which drug has found popularity in postoperative analgesia, especially in ambulatory surgery, because it does not cause drowsiness?

    a. Meperidine (Demerol)
    b. Ketorolac (Toradol)
    c. Diphenhydramine (Benadryl)
    d. Esmolol (Brevibloc)

22. Goserelin acetate implant (Zoladex) is a(n):

    a. Toxic chemotherapeutic agent
    b. Synthetic hormone
    c. Antihypertensive agent
    d. Anti-inflammatory drug

23. During a colonoscopy, the physician appears to have difficulty advancing the colonoscope. Suddenly your patient cries out in pain. You are ready to prepare the patient for emergency surgery, because you suspect the patient has suffered a:

    a. Gastric rupture
    b. Torn ligament
    c. Abscessed esophagus
    d. Perforated colon

24. During airway compromise, the nurse may be asked to assist by:

    a. Applying cricoid pressure
    b. Placing the patient in trendelenburg position
    c. Intubating the patient
    d. Administering wet to dry soaks

25. Sudden spasmodic closure of the vocal cords is a(n):

    a. Muscle spasm
    b. Laryngospasm
    c. Dysthymia
    d. Gastric reflex

# INTRODUCTION

As the delivery of health care undergoes major reform and revolution in America, so does the way in which that care is delivered to the patient. Fueled by soaring health care costs, this trend directs that patients will be treated not on an inpatient, but on an ambulatory basis. Indeed, one estimate is that 60% of primary care will be delivered on an ambulatory basis in the 1990s (Yale, 1993 AORN April 57:4 p. 901). Invasive procedures that just ten years ago would have been performed on hospitalized patients are now conducted in ambulatory settings. As a result, nurses are finding themselves providing increasingly complex care to a wider variety of ambulatory patients. Cost containment is not the only factor influencing the trend to ambulatory care. Phenomenal advances in surgical techniques and anesthetic agents allow rapid recovery from surgery and other special procedures. A final factor in the movement to ambulatory care is the popularity and satisfaction with the system expressed by both patients and their health care practitioners. Nurses can expect to see more surgical and special procedures performed on an ambulatory basis because of these four developments. This trend will impact clinical nursing practices because it will expand the nurse's responsibilities. It will also require refined nursing skills and enhanced knowledge of the special needs of ambulatory patients.

When initially conceived earlier this century, ambulatory care was targeted at the healthy patient, but that concept has since evolved dramatically. In the 1990s, patients who are in poor health may be admitted as ambulatory patients for same day surgery or other diagnostic and therapeutic procedures. Heightened interest in cost control now means that third party payers such as Medicare, Medicaid, and private insurers often make the final decision on whether a patient will be treated as ambulatory or inpatient. While this situation generally raises frustration in health care professionals and patients themselves, it is most likely here to stay.

The purpose of this book is to explore this trend in nursing: ambulatory patient care. Whether you're working in a physician's office, a walk-in medical clinic, a freestanding ambulatory facility, or the ambulatory department of a major hospital, you can expect to provide nursing care to ambulatory patients in increasing numbers during your career.

This book is designed as an overview of the various aspects of ambulatory patient care; this book reviews essential aspects of the clinical nursing care of the ambulatory patient and offers guidelines for planning care and nursing intervention for the ambulatory patient. After completing this book, you should have an increased awareness of common needs and nursing diagnoses of ambulatory patients. You should be able to begin plannning care and intervention for the many types of ambulatory patients you will encounter in your nursing practice.

Ambulatory nursing is an exciting new specialty on the cutting edge of twenty-first century health care. This is a field in its infancy that will experience explosive growth this decade. And it is a field that will need nurses who have the essential skills required to deliver ambulatory patient care.

# CHAPTER 1

# THE REVOLUTION IN AMBULATORY PATIENT CARE

## CHAPTER OBJECTIVE

After reading this chapter, you should have an increased awareness of changes in the delivery of health care that have occurred this century, how those changes have led to increased utilization of ambulatory care, and what to expect in future trends in ambulatory patient care.

## LEARNING OBJECTIVES

After reading this chapter, you should be able to:

1. Indicate factors in health care that led to the increased utilization of ambulatory services.

2. Recognize the definition of ambulatory care.

3. Differentiate between advantages and disadvantages of ambulatory care.

4. Identify trends that are expected to influence ambulatory care in the future.

## INTRODUCTION

Fueled by soaring health care costs, insurers (including the federal and state governments) are encouraging and even dictating that many types of health care will be delivered on an ambulatory basis. This results in a higher volume and broader variety of procedures being performed on patients who may be in less than optimal health. It is this broadening scope of ambulatory care, plus the fact that such care is no longer restricted to patients who are ideal candidates for ambulatory procedures, that poses a challenge to today's nurse.

This chapter scans ambulatory patient care: past, present and future. After reading this chapter, you should have an increased awareness of the changes in the delivery of health care that occurred this century, how those changes led to increased utilization of ambulatory care, and future trends that may develop in this field.

# THE DEVELOPMENT OF AMBULATORY SERVICES

Ambulatory care is defined here as the delivery of a health care service to a patient who is admitted for the day to receive that care and then is discharged that same day. Please note that the patient need not actually be ambulatory or walking under his or her own power to receive ambulatory care as it is defined here. In fact, physically impaired patients are routinely treated as ambulatory patients. For example, a paraplegic might have a cystoscopy, or an elderly woman confined to a wheelchair may have a cataract extraction in the ambulatory surgery department. The care the ambulatory patient receives may be diagnostic, such as a myelogram, or therapeutic, such as surgery or chemotherapy.

The concept of ambulatory care or outpatient treatment is not new to nurses. Ambulatory patient care programs have been in place at some health care institutions for over 25 years. However, it is interesting to note that even early in this century some health care professionals were advocating that patients be treated on an ambulatory basis: in 1918, the first general anesthetic was administered for ambulatory surgery. In the 1940s, the benefits of early ambulation were described, and in 1961, what is believed to be the first ambulatory surgery program in this country was launched at Butterworth Hospital in Michigan (Burden, 1993 p. 4,5). A "Come and Go" Surgery Unit opened at George Washington University in Washington, D. C. in 1966, as did an Outpatient Clinic at UCLA in California (Gruendemann & Meeker, 1987 p. 180). The first freestanding ambulatory surgery facility opened in Phoenix, Arizona in 1970 (Burden, 1993 p. 5).

When initially conceived earlier this century, the concept of ambulatory care was targeted at the healthy patient. This patient was generally healthy with no significant medical problems other than perhaps the one that the patient sought treatment for. It was assumed that these young healthy patients would be the ones offered the alternative of ambulatory care, while patients who were in less than optimal health would continue to receive their care in hospitals. That concept has since evolved dramatically, and therein lies the challenge for most nurses.

Ambulatory care proved both popular and successful as healthy patients flowed through the system. Nurses liked the emphasis on wellness and the promotion of self care; physicians and patients appreciated the convenience of ambulatory care that was generally free of tedious hospital routines and paperwork. Insurers were quick to note that ambulatory procedures reduced hospitalization costs, and thus cost became a significant factor in the decision to utilize ambulatory care. Faced with soaring health care costs, insurers began to insist that many procedures be performed on an ambulatory basis; patients who declined could be responsible for the increased cost of non-ambulatory care. This meant that patients who in the past would not have been considered candidates for ambulatory care started showing up on ambulatory procedure schedules around the country.

With this trend towards ambulatory care becoming an accepted standard, health care providers met the challenge by developing technology that refined and facilitated ambulatory care. Technological advances included the use of endoscopic instruments such as arthroscopes and laparoscopes that reduced or eliminated the need for large incisions and surgical explorations through tissue. Laser technology reduced tissue trauma and shortened surgical time. As physicians refined their skills in these techniques, a number of surgical and diagnostic or therapeutic procedures were shifted from inpatient to ambulatory status. Orthopedics and gynecology are two of the many specialties that underwent major transformation due to the advances in surgical technology. For example, a number of knee injuries that a decade ago might have meant an extensive surgical procedure and hospitalization are now corrected through an arthroscope on ambulatory patients.

These developments in surgical technology meant patients would have less tissue trauma and smaller incisions, which in turn meant more procedures could be performed on an ambulatory basis. So returning patients to their homes the same day made short-acting anesthetic agents essential. Having patients alert and street-ready within a matter of hours after anesthesia had never before been essential. Now anesthetists were faced with the need for anesthetic agents that would provide adequate analgesia and anesthesia, but which allowed a rapid return to consciousness and coherence. Several such drugs have debuted in just the past few years; their use has transformed anesthetic care of the ambulatory patient. More information about these new drugs can be found in Chapter 5.

Despite technologic and pharmacologic advances, ambulatory patient care still faces serious challenges. The ideal ambulatory patient is one who is free of significant medical disease and who has a support person at home who is able to meet his or her needs postoperatively. However, this is not always the case. Nurses providing care to ambulatory patients are often finding these patients in less than optimum condition and lacking in adequate support at home. For example, when an elderly man undergoes ambulatory surgery, his frail, elderly wife may be the only one at home to provide him with assistance during his recovery.

Those who pay the patient's bills, such as the government or private insurers, usually consider ambulatory care to be a cost-effective alternative. In fact, ambulatory care is no longer as often an alternative as it is a dictum. Unless patients can pay the bills themselves, they may have no choice other than to abide by their insurer's instructions. Large insurers may employ physicians or nurses who will review a specific patient's circumstances and make a recommendation on a case by case basis, but their opinion is not always consistent with the opinion of the professionals caring for the patient. The result is a patient admitted for ambulatory care who would not have been considered a candidate for ambulatory care even a few years ago.

Another interesting aspect of the health care reform movement is the decision of some insurers and the government to evaluate facilities on the quality of care provided. The parameters measured to assess facilities include mortality and morbidity rates along with costs and lengths of stay for common diagnoses. Facilities also may be evaluated on how efficiently their equipment is used and how efficiently care is delivered that is, how quickly patients can be moved through the system without negatively affecting outcomes. Facilities that do not fare well on these measures may experience a loss or decrease in reimbursement or face closing. Because nurses influence each of these aspects, they exert tremendous influence on the outcomes. So the quality of nursing care can not only influence the patient's health, but alter the health care institution's future.

# AMBULATORY CARE: ADVANTAGES & DISADVANTAGES

As with anything in life, ambulatory care has its advantages and its disadvantages: one size does not fit all. The following is a list of some of the advantages and disadvantages of ambulatory care (Chitwood & Swain, 1992 p. 109).

### Advantages

Advantages of ambulatory care generally address areas of cost and convenience, but also reflect patient care:

- **Cost:** Ambulatory care is generally less expensive and more cost efficient than inpatient hospital care.

- **Early discharge:** The hazards of immobility, especially after surgery, have been well documented. Ambulatory care emphasizes a return to a familiar environment as soon as is possible and desirable. The risk of nosocomial infections is reduced in ambulatory care, as is anxiety in many patients.

- **Patient and staff satisfaction:** Ambulatory care is generally more efficient and usually involves less paperwork than inpatient care. Patients often receive their care in or near the area where they check-in, and they generally express overall satisfaction with ambulatory care. Physicians appreciate the convenience for their patients, getting the procedures done efficiently, and not having to make hospital rounds. Nurses often have more opportunities to provide personalized care in the more informal ambulatory setting.

- **Emphasis on wellness:** Ambulatory care requires the patient and his or her support person to participate in certain aspects of care, with the emphasis on returning the patient to the highest possible level of pre-procedure functioning. This means the patient must learn more about his or her illness, and it also reduces patient dependency.

### Disadvantages

Disadvantages of ambulatory care generally reflect issues of efficiency and patient care.

- **Efficiency:** Health care facilities are increasingly examining the efficiency with which care is delivered while insurers are limiting the fees paid for these services, so nurses and patients sometimes find themselves caught in the middle of a battle between quality care and cost-efficient care. The emphasis on efficiency in ambulatory procedures can potentially dehumanize the patient's care, and ambulatory care nurses can be stressed to the point of burnout by the haste with which the nursing process (assessment, diagnosis, planning, implementation, and evaluation) must be completed. Nurses in ambulatory care are also responsible for teaching the patient and his or her support person about postoperative care, care that would be provided by a nurse in an inpatient setting.

- **Patient care:** Some patients are not good candidates for ambulatory care because of medical illness or their support person's inability to insure adequate aftercare at home.

# ALTERNATIVES TO AMBULATORY CARE

With insurers pushing many diagnostic, therapeutic and surgical procedures from the inpatient to ambulatory arena, health care providers have sought solutions to their dilemma. One solution is the genesis of extended observation or overnight care in the facility. Insurers will often still pay for this as ambulatory care and the patient and family benefit from not having to accept responsibility for care that is beyond their ability to deliver. "Short stay" surgery helps bridge the gap between some surgeries that are too complex to allow patient discharge the same day and those that really do not require typical inpatient hospital care; some ambulatory facilities can care for patients up to 72 hours postoperatively. Nurses can generally expect to see more procedures shifted in this manner in the future (Llewellyn, 1991 p. 1179 AORN May, 53:5).

Another alternative is the development of "medical" hotels and assisted-care facilities. These are facilities that are separate from the place where ambulatory care was received, but often are located near the health care facility. This is a type of step down unit or transitional unit for patients who undergo an ambulatory procedure but who do not feel ready to return home. Patients in these areas may have an attendant or assistant who can assist them as they recover. This may or may not be covered by their insurer.

# THE FUTURE OF AMBULATORY CARE

Whether you're a nurse working in a physician's office, a walk-in medical clinic, a freestanding ambulatory facility, or the ambulatory department of a major hospital, you can expect to provide care to ambulatory patients in increasing numbers during your career. Because health care reform is underway but incomplete, it is impossible to say what the future will hold for ambulatory care. It does seem probable that the trend to move patient care from an inpatient sector to an ambulatory basis will continue and strengthen. Nurses can expect that their responsibilities will also increase consistent with this trend. However, it is also reasonable to assume that technology will continue to advance and provide exciting alternatives to inpatient care. The bottom line seems to be that while the specialty of ambulatory health care is developing, it will be a nurse who puts it all together and insures that the caring never goes out of the care. Because insurers are dictating in some areas how patient care will be delivered, patients may begin to feel they are being treated more like a case number and less like a person. This is again an area where nurses make the difference. The following will be some of the challenges for the ambulatory patient care nurse:

- Complete the nursing process to deliver safe and efficient care within a time frame that spans only hours, rather than days (as with an inpatient).

- Preserve the patient's dignity and privacy in an area that is deliberately condensed to increase efficiency.

- Insure that the patient feels he or she is being treated with respect as a person and does not feel like a case to be moved through the system as quickly as possible.

- Teach the patient and/or support person(s) the skills and knowledge that will be required to provide postoperative carecare that hospitalized patients would generally receive from their nurse. This will require the nurse to have skill in both written and verbal interpersonal communication and teaching.

- Return the patient to his or her support person or residence as quickly as is safe and practical.

# SUMMARY

This chapter briefly reviewed the past, present, and expected future of ambulatory care. The history of ambulatory care was discussed. Advances in technology and pharmacology and the subsequent influence on ambulatory care were discussed. General patient and staff satisfaction with ambulatory care was noted. The fact that insurers (including the federal and state governments) are encouraging and even dictating that many types of health care will be delivered on an ambulatory basis was discussed. The broadening scope of ambulatory care plus the fact that such care is no longer restricted to patients who are ideal candidates for ambulatory procedures was covered. The challenges for nurses who care for ambulatory patients were presented.

# CRITICAL CONCEPTS

- The decision to treat a person as an ambulatory patient rather than as an inpatient is often made by the patient's insurer.

- Advances in technology such as the arthroscope and laparoscope facilitated the development of ambulatory surgery.

- Pharmacologic developments in anesthesia facilitated the utilization of ambulatory surgery.

- Nurses who provide ambulatory patient care must be efficient, caring, and skilled in interpersonal communication and patient teaching.

- It is likely that the trend towards treating patients in ambulatory settings will continue and such utilization will probably increase in the future.

# EXAM QUESTIONS

## Chapter 1

Questions 1-4

1. Factors that led to the increased utilization of ambulatory care include all except:

    a. patient preference
    b. insurer's decisions
    c. physician satisfaction with ambulatory care
    d. development of long acting anesthetic agents ✓

2. All of these patients would likely be classified as ambulatory except:

    a. a paraplegic male coming for cystoscopy
    b. a multigravida admitted for elective cesarean xection ✓
    c. a wheelchair-bound elderly female having cataract extraction
    d. a young male having arthroscopic knee surgery

3. Disadvantages of ambulatory care can include:

    a. pressure on the nurse to complete the nursing process in a short time frame ✓
    b. decreased cost to the patient
    c. increased utilization of the facility
    d. enhanced and advanced care delivery to the patient

4. Alternatives to ambulatory care can include:

    a. admission to a hospital's critical care area
    b. a 23-hour stay after an ambulatory procedure ✓
    c. keeping the patient in the Recovery Room for 16 hours
    d. asking the family to provide bedside care in the hospital

# CHAPTER 2

# THE AMBULATORY PATIENT CARE FACILITY

## CHAPTER OBJECTIVE

After completing this chapter, you should be better prepared to distinguish between the different types of facilities where ambulatory patient care is provided, describe the relative advantages and disadvantages of each, and recognize how the different types of facilities may influence nursing practice.

## LEARNING OBJECTIVES

After reading this chapter, you should be able to:

1. Differentiate between types of facilities where ambulatory patient care is offered.

2. Specify the potential advantages and disadvantages of each different type of ambulatory facility.

3. Choose nursing actions for prevention and intervention of selected non-medical emergencies.

4. Recognize how the different types of facilities may influence nursing practice.

## INTRODUCTION

Ambulatory patient care is delivered in a wide variety of different facilities, from hospitals to freestanding centers to physician offices. The purpose of this chapter is to give you an overview of the different types of facilities where ambulatory patient care may be delivered, and some of the relative advantages and disadvantages of each. Basic nursing considerations for practice in each of these facilities will be reviewed, and the issue of standards of care for ambulatory facilities will be briefly addressed. The environment, disaster preparation, and security at the ambulatory facility will be briefly surveyed with the emphasis on nursing responsibilities. The chapter closes with a summary and a review of the critical concepts presented.

## TYPES OF AMBULATORY PATIENT CARE FACILITIES

As noted in Chapter 1, there is a nationwide trend towards providing patient care on an ambulatory rather than an inpatient basis. This trend is fueled largely by third party payers such as the government or insurance companies. These agencies often will determine whether their insured patient will be treated on an ambulatory basis, and if so, where that care will be delivered: in a hospital, physician's office, or freestanding facility. The insurance company usually bases these decisions on examination of the costs and evaluations of the quality of care delivered by available ambulatory facilities within the community. Facilities that can demonstrate delivery of cost effective yet high quality care will be strategically positioned for the future. Cost effectiveness is usually measured against other similar facilities in the area. Quality of care may be measured by expected patient outcomes, patient satisfaction with the care, and mortality and morbidity rates. In some areas, insurers or businesses form consortiums to evaluate health care providers and facilities. Then these groups will negotiate reduced health care fees and in return agree to send their patients to these facilities and providers. It should be clear then that whoever is paying the bill for the care will have significant influence on where that care is delivered.

Although at times it seems to defy logic, insurers and government programs sometimes will reimburse for a procedure only when it is performed in a specific setting but not another, regardless of the actual cost. But where ambulatory care is received is not often as important to most patients as the convenience and quality of that care and the manner in which it is delivered. As we approach the close of this century, we are seeing patients with heightened consumer awareness. This means patients themselves are evaluating facilities, asking about accreditation (as in mammography clinics) and checking on costs. But regardless of who is asking the questions, who is paying the bill, and where the care is delivered, all patients have the right to expect quality care.

The different types of facilities where ambulatory patient care is delivered each have relative but not absolute advantages and disadvantages. Below you'll find described three common types facilities: hospitals, freestanding centers, and physician offices. The relative advantages and disadvantages of each and the implications for nurses providing patient care at these facilities are briefly mentioned below.

## Hospitals

With patients being lost to convenient freestanding centers and sophisticated physician office clinics, hospitals countered by developing ambulatory departments within their own systems. In some cases, a hospital dedicates a part of the existing facility to ambulatory patient care. This may simply be a separate area for admission and discharge, or the patient may actually receive the ambulatory care in this special unit. Some hospitals construct freestanding facilities to treat their ambulatory patients while still utilizing their main facility for support services such as maintenance and billing.

- Advantages: Because of the wealth of support services and specialists on staff, it would seem that hospitals are better equipped to manage emergencies, although there is no documentation to support this claim (Burden, 1993 p. 19). If an ambulatory patient must be admitted, the transfer can be completed with a minimum of travel and difficulty. Obviously, hospitals have significant purchasing power that many small clinics do not. And with administrative services already in place, there is no need for duplication of staff and personnel for a separate facility.

- Disadvantages: Hospitals are renowned as impersonal bureaucracies mired in red tape. Professional staff and technology are expensive, and so hospital costs can be higher. Dissatisfaction often surges when ambulatory patients find themselves funnelled into a tedious and time consuming inpatient system.

- Nursing considerations: The ambulatory patient care nurse working in a hospital may be frustrated by the paperwork and regulations inherent in a hospital environment. Getting skilled help in an emergency in a hospital should theoretically be easier than getting help in a freestanding facility or doctor's office, because those helpers must journey to the facility once notification of an emergency is given. Because a hospital is open 24 hours a day, the nurse working here may not feel quite as pressured to rush the ambulatory patient out in time for closing; that is, the patient can be transferred to an inpatient unit if necessary. In a freestanding clinic, the patient must go by ambulance or other form of special patient transport if hospital admission is necessary.

## Freestanding Units

The explosive growth in the number of freestanding ambulatory patient care facilities is a testimony to the success of these diagnostic and therapeutic facilities. Many of these clinics are operated efficiently with a small staff and are therefore able to lower costs while increasing patient satisfaction. Some of these facilities are dedicated to one therapeutic intervention such as surgery, chemotherapy, dialysis, or physical therapy. Others may be limited to diagnostics such as radiologic exams. A recent phenomenon is the development of urgent care or minor emergency clinics. Patients without primary care physicians turn to these facilities when they need care for anything from flu to an ankle sprain.

- Advantages: Convenience and cost-effective care are hallmarks of the freestanding center. Usually small, these facilities are often able to offer more personal attention to the patient; patients may feel less overwhelmed or anxious than they would in a large hospital. Paperwork is often reduced and families are often able to remain with the patient longer in freestanding facilities. Recent nursing research indicated patient satisfaction was greater when ambulatory surgery was performed in a freestanding center as opposed to a hospital-based unit (Pica-Furey, 1993 AORN J 57:5 May, p. 1119-1127). Patients in this study expressed greater satisfaction with the convenience and cost of care as well as the courtesy of the staff.

- Disadvantages: Whether warranted or not, many believe that a hospital may be better prepared to manage emergencies and critical situations. This is the reason that patients who are in poor health or who are high-risk for complications may be referred to a hospital-based facility rather than a freestanding unit when ambulatory care is required.

- Nursing considerations: The freestanding unit often offers nurses an unparalleled opportunity to practice the nursing process and to utilize a wide variety of nursing skills in doing so. However, the nurse employed in a facility other than a hospital may be expected to shoulder additional responsibilities in the absence of a support staff. Because the staff is generally limited in number, nurses working in these units must often be quite versatile and flexible in filling different positions. For example, duties of the freestanding surgery unit nurse may include scrubbing for the operation, recovering the patient from anesthesia, and dispensing drugs for discharge. Also, in some freestanding units nurses may find themselves left in the building without physician support as they care for a patient not quite ready for discharge.

## Physician offices

The physician's office has long been a major facility for ambulatory patient care. However, reimbursement issues are now clouding the situation. In some cases, physicians find they will not be reimbursed for certain procedures performed in their offices; in others, the care will not be covered unless it is received in the office. How physician office practices will be affected by proposed health care reform remains to be seen.

- Advantages: Convenient for the patient and generally cost-effective for the patient and insurer, a number of physician's offices are even equipped to perform advanced procedures such as surgery. Podiatrists, plastic surgeons, and ophthalmologists are common providers of this type of sophisticated in-office care.

- Disadvantages: Technology is expensive and not all physicians will be able to invest in the equipment and staff necessary to meet standards of care and support patient safety; reimbursement for in-office procedures may vary or be limited.

- Nursing considerations: While the physician's office may offer the nurse an opportunity for more direct patient contact and care, the office nurse also is often distracted by a number of other responsibilities including administrative tasks.

# STANDARDS FOR AMBULATORY PATIENT CARE FACILITIES

Ambulatory patients have the right to expect that certain standards of care will be met, regardless of where that care is delivered. Appendix A includes addresses of two national professional organizations that evaluate and accredit certain ambulatory care facilities: Accreditation Association for Ambulatory Health Care and the Joint Commission for Accreditation of Health Care Organizations. The ambulatory facility should also meet local building and health codes. Specialty care facilities may be inspected and certified by their specialty organization; an example is mammography centers, which may be accredited by the American College of Radiology.

# THE AMBULATORY CARE FACILITY

Regardless of the type of ambulatory care facility, there are specific concerns nurses caring for ambulatory patients should consider when planning that care.

## The environment

Like any other patient care environment, the ambulatory facility should focus on the patient's needs first. Below are listed some nursing considerations for the ambulatory patient care facility:

- Segregate patients being prepared for a procedure from those recovering from a procedure, because seeing postoperative patients bandaged or vomiting may distress the preoperative patient.

- Guard patient privacy; conduct interviews out of hearing range of other patients. Privacy is a fundamental right of the patient even in the confines of a small ambulatory facility.

- Respect patient dignity to help increase patient comfort and confidence in the facility and staff. For example, the patient should not be led through the facility holding a thin gown shut in the back with one hand and clutching her clothes in the other hand.

- Minimize the number of stops (laboratory, radiology, business office) a patient has to make before the procedure; this helps reduce stress.

- Allow the patient's support person to remain with him or her until the procedure begins if the patient so desires; this may help reduce anxiety.

- Consider providing refreshments, reading matter, or television for those waiting on the patient; this can help reduce their anxiety. Access to a telephone is always welcomed; separate play areas for children may prove helpful.

It is also appropriate to note that the nurse's safety is also essential. Even small facilities must provide the nurse with appropriate barrier protection such as eye shields and masks when indicated, or other protective gear like lead aprons to reduce exposure to radiation.

### Disaster preparation

Most hospital-based nurses remember receiving instruction in disaster preparation during their orientation to the facility. Hospitals generally have extensive disaster plans; freestanding ambulatory units and physician's offices should also have firm plans in place. Nurses working in freestanding facilities should review and learn the disaster plan for their facility, because there will be fewer resource people such as security personnel to rely upon in the event of a real disaster. The following strategies should help reduce risk and potential mortality and morbidity:

- Develop a mental plan at the beginning of each work day for responding to a fire in your area; know the location of a fire extinguisher and how to use it. Know how to call the fire department, and what to do until help arrives. More than one person on the staff should know how to shut off oxygen to the facility, because oxygen can fuel a fire.

- Formulate a contingency plan for meeting the challenges of a devastating storm such as a tornado.

- Plan and practice for an earthquake if you live in an earthquake risk zone.

- Develop a bomb threat plan; know who to call in this situation.

### Security

While hospital-based units are usually able to call upon a security guard or staff when needed, many small freestanding facilities do not employ security officers. Yet these centers may be vulnerable to crime because they are businesses with controlled drugs and cash on the premises. The following strategies may reduce risk:

- Keep prescription pads and drugs locked up and do not discuss with patients or others the types and amounts of drugs stored on the premises.

- Do not leave cash out on desks; insure that every staff member knows how to call for police and emergency help.

- Be aware of your surroundings; report suspicious people.

Note that responsibility for patient safety also may involve reporting to the authorities and seeking resources when you suspect your ambulatory patient may have been a victim of a crime such as child abuse or spouse abuse. Check your state's laws to learn your specific obligations, but be aware that aside from the ethical concerns, liability could result from returning an injured ambulatory patient to the abuser after treatment for injuries.

# SUMMARY

The purpose of this chapter was to give you an overview of the different types of facilities where ambulatory patient care may be delivered, and some of the potential advantages and disadvantages of each. Nursing considerations for practice in each of these facilities was reviewed, and the issue of standards of care was briefly addressed. The environment, disaster preparation, and security at the ambulatory facility were also discussed in the context of nursing responsibilities.

# CRITICAL CONCEPTS

- Reimbursement is often the key issue in determining where ambulatory care will be delivered.

- Quality of care (as measured by patient outcomes, mortality and morbidity, and patient satisfaction) and cost-effectiveness are two essential parameters used to evaluate ambulatory facilities.

- Patients have the right to expect that an ambulatory facility will meet certain standards of care regardless of size; national organizations can inspect and accredit many ambulatory facilities.

- Hospitals offering ambulatory services draw upon relatively vast resources when providing that care; freestanding facilities generally have fewer resources but may be able to provide more personal attention and convenience to the patient.

- Patient rights, including privacy and dignity, must be upheld even in a small facility where patients are in close quarters.

- Disastrous events such as fires are easier prevented than treated, so the ambulatory care nurse should know how to prevent these incidents but also what to do if one occurs.

# EXAM QUESTIONS
## Chapter 2

Questions 5-7

5. Ambulatory facilities can be inspected and accredited by the:

    a. accreditation Association for Ambulatory Health Care
    b. joint Commission on Ambulatory Health Care
    c. national Organization of Nurses
    d. physician's Accreditation Committee for Ambulatory Care

6. A future trend in ambulatory care may include:

    a. denial of care to patients who do not comply with instructions
    b. strictly limiting ambulatory services to healthy patients
    c. asking patients to provide their own meals and medications
    d. accepting sicker patients for ambulatory procedures

7. As providers of ambulatory care, hospitals have the advantage of:

    a. greater resources
    b. less paperwork
    c. easy access
    d. lower cost

# CHAPTER 3

# THE NURSING PROCESS AND THE AMBULATORY PATIENT

## CHAPTER OBJECTIVE

After reading this chapter, you should be better prepared to recognize the steps of the nursing process and identify how that process may be shaped by the special needs of the ambulatory patient.

## LEARNING OBJECTIVES

After reading this chapter, you should be able to:

1. Recognize the five components of the nursing process.

2. Differentiate between distinct needs of the ambulatory patient versus the inpatient.

3. Specify common adaptations in the nursing care plan that may be indicated based on the unique concerns of the ambulatory patient.

4. Indicate specific considerations that are unique to the ambulatory patient's care.

## INTRODUCTION

Most nurses remember the tedious hours spent writing care plans during their training programs, but many subsequently give only cursory attention to care plans after they begin professional practice. Most accreditation standards require some type of care plan for each patient, so something resembling a care plan can usually be found on a patient's chart. This may simply be a standardized care plan printed out by the computer and placed on the patient's chart by the unit secretary. Despite this, most nurses should know that practical, feasible plans for patient care are essential to professional nursing practice because they facilitate nursing care and document the nursing process. This chapter will review the nursing process and describe how it is shaped by the special needs of the ambulatory patient. Care plans will be reviewed and their practical clinical application in ambulatory patient care will be discussed. The chapter briefly addresses some of the issues pertinent to ambulatory patient care such as standards of care, advance directives, and the patient's rights. The chapter closes with a summary and a list of the critical concepts presented.

# AMBULATORY CARE AND THE NURSING PROCESS

Every day nurses assess their patients in order to plan and implement skilled nursing care. Nurses can then evaluate their care based on expected patient outcomes. This process generally runs smoothly and the patient receives professional nursing care that moves him closer to his highest possible level of wellness; both nurse and patient express satisfaction with the care delivered and received. Nevertheless, physicians and patients often still perceive that all nurses do is carry out the doctor's orders. An erroneous assumption that minimizes and denigrates the value of professional nursing care, this misconception must be combatted directly by practicing nurses. One way to dispel the notion that all nurses do is carry out doctor's orders is to utilize and document the nursing process, including a fifth component recently incorporated into the process: nursing diagnosis. When nurses document their care, their contribution to the patient's health care and impact on the outcome is clear. Professional respect and autonomy are the result.

Using the nursing process to plan care should not simply be an empirical exercise. The nursing process and care plans you studied during training really do have practical application in clinical care. In fact, in ambulatory care, using the nursing process can facilitate patient care. Because the nursing process must be compressed into a period of hours rather days or months, ambulatory patient care is a specialty especially amenable to the use of the nursing process. One reason is that the nursing process helps you get organized. These systematic steps are easy to remember, and with practice you will find that using the nursing process enhances your ability to deliver consistent quality patient care. This is because you use the system to guide you in patient care, rather than approaching each of your patients as an assortment of needs. Using the nursing process enables you to work more efficiently and set priorities in your care giving. Efficient time management is an essential characteristic of ambulatory care nurses because of the compressed time frame for care. Using the nursing process not only helps you get organized, it helps you deliver quality care more consistently and documents the value of your nursing care: you're doing more than just carrying out the doctor's orders.

The nursing process encompasses five steps: assessment, diagnosis, planning, implementation, and evaluation. Many nurses recall four steps, but you should note that in recent years a fifth component, diagnosis, was added. All five steps of the nursing process are reviewed below. This review is designed to help you learn to adapt the nursing process to ambulatory patient care. It is not comprehensive discussion, because that can be found in textbooks on the subject.

## Assessment

Gathering information about the patient is the first step of the nursing process. Assessment data comes from the patient's history, the physical examination, and laboratory studies (Sparks & Taylor, 1991 p. 1). An accurate assessment is the key to effective nursing process, because it forms the foundation upon which the whole process is built. Experienced nurses find that practice builds skill in patient assessment; assessment skills are essential in ambulatory patient care because nurses are making decisions about the patient, such as readiness for discharge, based on this assessment. A textbook on physical examination can help you refine your physical assessment skills.

## Diagnosis

The North American Nursing Diagnosis Association (NANDA) defines nursing diagnosis as a "clinical judgment about individual, family, or community responses to actual or potential health problems or to life processes. Nursing diagnosis provide the basis for selection of nursing interventions to achieve outcomes for which the nurse is accountable." A nursing diagnoses often includes problems or potential problems and the aspects that the nurse can independently act upon.(Sparks & Taylor, 1991 p. 10). You select this nursing diagnosis based on the information you gathered during your assessment of the patient. While the concept of nursing diagnosis may not be familiar to all nurses, it is an indispensable one. This second step of the nursing process draws on all your skills as a nurse and develops your professional autonomy. In addition, patient care is enhanced by identifying potential problems before they occur and by focusing not just on the patient's disease, but on his whole being: mind, body and spirit. A reference text listing nursing diagnoses is an invaluable aid for this step of the nursing process and will expedite care planning. Chapters later in this book will present common nursing diagnoses for selected groups of patients and common nursing actions for those diagnoses.

## Planning

Once the nursing diagnosis is made, the planning of care can begin. According to Sparks& Taylor (1991 p. 15), planning involves four stages:

- Assigning priorities: This guides you to focus on high-priority concerns first. For example, an ineffective breathing pattern is clearly a higher priority than a knowledge deficit.

- Establishing expected outcomes: Setting goals helps you determine what you expect to accomplish with your nursing care and forms the basis for evaluating your progress.

- Selecting nursing actions: With the diagnoses made and the goals selected, this phase helps you determine which nursing interventions will most likely be effective in reaching the expected outcomes.

- Documentation: In this phase you commit to the patient's record the steps of the nursing process. Putting it in writing is critical in staff communication and may be a deciding factor in the event your care is challenged (Kemmy, 1993 AORN April, 57:4, p. 958). In some cases, especially Medicare, reimbursement may be dependent upon documentation.

## Implementation

As you go to work, your nursing care is directed at the problems or potential problems you have identified. In ambulatory care, implementation usually includes the patient's support person or family; this generally involves teaching them about home care and potential complications that may develop after they leave the ambulatory unit. Nurses providing care to ambulatory patients therefore require interpersonal communication and teaching skills.

## Evaluation

As the final step in the nursing process, evaluation examines the outcome of your care. During the evaluation process, you determine if your patient is meeting the outcomes you expected. Based on this information, you continue care or redirect your intervention as needed. In ambulatory patient care, parts of this evaluation often take the form of a follow up telephone call, since the patient will be discharged the same day. Evaluation may also mean assessing the support person's ability to provide care. In cases such as ambulatory surgery, the support person will often be expected to provide care such as observation or medication administration that would be performed by a nurse if the patient were hospitalized. Evaluation also validates the value of nursing care as confirmed by the positive outcomes.

Clearly, the five steps of the nursing process guide and facilitate nursing care. The process becomes even more valuable in ambulatory patient care, when there is less time to accomplish goals and return patients to their highest possible level of functioning.

Within this nursing process are some challenges that are specific to ambulatory care as opposed to inpatient care. Those include the compressed time frame for care and the fact that a support person may be the provider of post-procedure care, rather than a nurse. This will require teaching by a nurse who has good communication skills. Some of the ways that ambulatory nursing differs from inpatient nursing are described below:

- The ambulatory nurse generally cares for patients of all ages, from infants to the elderly. The inpatient nurse usually cares either for adults, children, or the elderly, because he or she is frequently assigned to a specific floor or area of the hospital where there is little mixing if these patients.

- The ambulatory nurse's patients often present with a wide variety of medical and surgical disorders; the inpatient nurse's patients generally fall in similar specialties, such as orthopedics, cardiology, or neurology.

- The ambulatory nurse generally only has an opportunity to assess the patient immediately before the procedure; the inpatient nurse will often be able to assess the patient hours or even a day or more before a scheduled procedure.

- Teaching of the ambulatory patient begins upon the patient's arrival, continues throughout the procedure, and involves teaching not only the patient but also the person who will be providing home care. Inpatient nurses often do not begin formal discharge planning and teaching until the physician writes an order for discharge.

- The final step of the nursing process, evaluation, often is only finally completed over the telephone, because the patient is discharged that same day. Inpatient nurses usually are able to evaluate the outcome of their care at the patient's bedside.

Burden (1993 p. 110) also identified some of the unique responsibilities of the ambulatory surgery nurse:

Ultimate patient outcome for the ambulatory surgery population is greatly affected by nursing decisions such as rapidity of initial attempts to ambulate or raise the patient's head, the timing and type of oral intake allowed, and the choice between several types or routes of medication ordered. Beyond this necessary attention to the patent's physiologic needs, the nurse should recognize and address the patient's emotional, cultural, and spiritual needs and promote the patient's dignity and privacy at all times. The fact that there is no nurse "on the next shift", when a patient returns home, requires an exacting thoroughness from the nurse in the ambulatory surgery facility. That often means spending a significant amount of time providing instructions to the patent and family and being involved in the details of the patient's transportation and home support needs (p. 110).

# SPECIAL CONSIDERATIONS IN AMBULATORY PATIENT CARE

Ambulatory care providers also need to be aware of some special issues involved in ambulatory care. These include standards of care, legal considerations, advance directives, and living wills.

## Standards of care

Different states have different requirements for building health care facilities; accrediting agencies also have standards that must be met. Most ambulatory facilities are expected to meet the same standards of care as other facilities where similar care takes place. In other words, the surgical care a patient receives in a freestanding ambulatory surgery center should be comparable to care that would be rendered in a hospital (Gruendemann & Meeker, 1987 p. 182). All aspects of care, such as nursing, anesthesia, and monitoring are expected to meet community standards. Patients sometimes do not realize this and are justifiably concerned that they may not receive quality care.

## Legal considerations

Ambulatory patients are usually assessed to be street-ready by their nurse, who generally notifies a physician of this readiness for discharge. The physician frequently accepts the nurse's assessment that the patient is ready to leave and may not personally examine the patient, so the nurse bears a considerable amount of responsibility for that assessment. Nearly all facilities require a patient who has received any sedation to be accompanied home by a responsible party. This is important because, if this patient harmed himself or others getting home, the nurse might be held liable. Releasing a patient to a support person who will continue their care at home also requires astute nursing assessment of that person's ability to provide the care. The nurse must be prepared to intervene if the support person expected to provide care does not seem capable of it; liability could result from releasing the patient to the care of a person unable meet their needs.

## Advance Directive

In 1990 Congress passed a law requiring that Medicare and Medicaid patients (St. Francis) be informed of their right to make choices about their treatment. This is known as Advance Directive Notification. Additional laws vary from one state to another on patient's rights and choices about care; you should familiarize yourself with these laws and your institution's policies.

## Patient rights and responsibility

The American Hospital Association has developed a statement of patient's rights; many institutions have added comments about the patient's responsibilities. In ambulatory care, these responsibilities may include an agreement to follow home care instructions and to provide a responsible adult for home care.

# SUMMARY

Practical, feasible plans for patient care are essential to professional nursing practice and ambulatory patient care because these plans facilitate nursing care and document the nursing process. This chapter reviewed the nursing process and describe how it is shaped by the special needs of the ambulatory patient. The chapter also addressed some of the issues unique to ambulatory patient care such as standards of care, advance directives, and patients' rights.

# CRITICAL CONCEPTS

- The nursing process facilitates and expedites nursing care of the ambulatory patient.

- The five steps of the nursing process are assessment, diagnosis, planning, implementation, and evaluation.

- Nursing diagnoses and evaluation of expected patient outcomes document the value of nursing care.

- Using and documenting the nursing process helps dispel the perception that nurses only carry out doctors' orders.

- Ambulatory patient care should not be of a lower standard than inpatient care for a similar procedure.

- Ambulatory nurses must be efficient time managers with sharp assessment skills and the ability to teach both the patient and support person.

# EXAM QUESTIONS

## Chapter 3

Questions 8-10

8. Ambulatory patient care is especially challenging to the nurse because of the:

   a. compressed time frame *(circled)*
   b. cost containment measures
   c. complex hospital admission forms
   d. tedious care plans

9. One difference between the inpatient and the ambulatory patient is the ambulatory patient's specific need for:

   a. discharge teaching *(circled)*
   b. oral hydration
   c. frequent turning
   d. heavy sedation

10. Assessment, diagnosis, planning, implementation and evaluation are components of the nursing:

    a. examination
    b. review
    c. intervention
    d. process *(circled)*

# CHAPTER 4

# SELECTION OF THE AMBULATORY PATIENT

## CHAPTER OBJECTIVE

After reading this chapter, you should be better prepared to discern which patients and procedures are ideally suited to ambulatory care, which are more appropriately treated in an inpatient setting, and how that decision is influenced.

## LEARNING OBJECTIVES

After reading this chapter, you should be able to:

1. Differentiate between factors that influence the selection of patients for ambulatory vs. inpatient care.

2. Specify general guidelines that determine a patient's suitability for ambulatory care.

3. Indicate nursing actions that may influence the decision to treat the patient under alternative plans rather than ambulatory.

4. Identify the influence that third-party payers will have on the decision to provide ambulatory vs. inpatient care.

## INTRODUCTION

Proper patient selection is an essential aspect of the delivery of safe and effective ambulatory care. This chapter will describe how patients can be selected for ambulatory care and the types of procedures most amenable to the ambulatory setting. Patient selection based on age, health status, nature of the procedure, support system, physician, and third-party payers is reviewed. The final determination on ambulatory versus inpatient care is often made by a third-party payer. Ambulatory nurses must be prepared to meet this challenge and act as patient advocates when necessary. Considerations for the ambulatory patient care nurse are also presented. The chapter closes with a summary and a list of the critical concepts presented.

## SELECTING PATIENTS FOR AMBULATORY CARE

While ambulatory patients ideally are in good health with a strong support system, the reality is that more complex procedures are being performed on sicker patients. When ambulatory care was first conceived, the target population was healthy patients coming for short, relatively routine procedures. That scenario is constantly changing as an increasing number of procedures are pushed into the ambulatory care setting and even chronically ill or high-risk patients are admitted and discharged the same day. Some of these patients and procedures just ten years ago would have mandated hospitalization.

The criteria by which ambulatory patients now are selected is never static but dynamic and always changing. Major factors in the decision to care for a patient in the hospital versus an ambulatory unit are the patient's physician and the party paying for the procedure. As discussed in previous chapters, reimbursement is a key issue in determining where a diagnostic or therapeutic procedure will be performed; the physician's preference is also a significant factor. The following is a discussion of those factors and others that influence ambulatory patient selection. The other factors include age, health status, nature of the procedure, and support system. You should note that no clear standard exists for which patients are acceptable and which are not: this is heavily influenced by the type of facility where the procedure will take place, the skill and resources of those caring for the patient, and community standards. Below, you will find a simple review of some parameters that need to be considered when selecting patients for ambulatory care.

## Age

While the boundaries of age generally excluded the very young and the very old from ambulatory care in the past, age is seldom a deciding factor in selecting patients for ambulatory care today. However, age must be considered when it comes to the aftercare to be provided by a support person or family member. That person must be capable of providing care after dischargecare that in the hospitalized patient would be provided by a nurse. So the elderly patient may require additional support at home for aftercare or the funds for private duty care in the home or residence. Also, some infants born prematurely or with a history of apnea are thought to require careful monitoring at home or hospital admission for observation. However, in general, age is seldom the sole deciding factor in patient selection for ambulatory care.

## Health status

The American Society of Anesthesiologists uses a system that classifies patient physical status (PS) before surgery; this is presented in Table 4-1.

Initially, ambulatory patients fell into the first two classifications; that has changed dramatically in the last decade. Now, patients in the PS 3 or even occasionally the PS 4 classification flow through ambulatory care units. A PS 2 classification patient could be one with well controlled mild hypertension who is otherwise healthy. Ideally, patients having an ambulatory procedure are healthy or only at low-risk for complications, like this patient. But this has all changed due to the influence of third-party payers and also as a result of technological advances. Simply put, ideal conditions seldom exist any longer. Physicians who prefer to treat a high-risk patient in the hospital rather than an ambulatory facility may be forced to debate the third-party payer for a negotiated decision.

Because ambulatory surgery patients are presenting with these increasingly complex histories, the patient is ideally assessed by the anesthetist and ambulatory nurse before the day of surgery. Additional blood tests or diagnostic studies can then be ordered and evaluated before the surgery; nursing assessment of the patient's support system and understanding of the ambulatory process can be completed. When patients arrive at the ambulatory facility only hours before their procedure, there may be inadequate time to secure these tests and surgery may be delayed. An example would be a patient on furosemide (Lasix) who needs to have a potassium level determined before general anesthesia or a patient with significant heart disease who needs to be evaluated by a cardiol-

# Table 4-1
## American Society of Anesthesiologists Physical Status (PS) Classifications

| | |
|---|---|
| PS 1 | A normal, healthy patient. |
| PS 2 | A patient with a mild systemic disease. Examples: patients with well controlled hypertension, diabetes controlled by diet or oral hypoglycemics, cigarette smokers. |
| PS 3 | A patient with severe systemic disease that limits activity. Examples: patients with heart disease and angina, severe asthma, complicated diabetes. |
| PS 4 | A patient with an incapacitating systemic disease that is a constant threat to life. Examples: patients with congestive heart failure, renal failure, uncontrolled angina pectoris, liver failure. |
| PS 5 | A moribund patient not expected to live without or with the operation. Examples: patients with ruptured aortic aneurysms, severe head injury, severe multiple trauma, embolus. |
| PS 6 | A patient who has been declared brain dead and is coming to surgery for harvesting of organs. |
| Emergency | The letter "E" is added to the classification if the operation is considered to be an emergency. |

ologist before undergoing the procedure. Patients sometimes resist this because of the inconvenience of two trips to the facility; this can prove a hardship to patients coming to the facility from out of town. In this case, the ambulatory facility's staff must rely upon the surgeon to order necessary tests and assess the patient's general suitability for ambulatory care. The ambulatory patient should also have the capacity to understand preoperative instructions such as NPO, or have available a support person who understands these instructions and can enforce them. These are critical points because failure to comply with pre-procedure instructions can alter the values of diagnostic tests and increase the risk of serious complications from anesthesia.

## Nature of the procedure

Before the debut of lasers and endoscopic procedures, surgery generally meant an incision and hospitalization. Technologic advances such as lasers have transformed many incisions into short puncture wounds; pharmacologic advances in anesthesia have revolutionized ambulatory care. This means that complex procedures which in the past would have required hospitalization are being performed on an ambulatory basis. Laparoscopic-assisted cholecystectomy and vaginal hysterectomy are two examples. Procedures that involve high risk of complications, long anesthetic times (usually more than 4 hours), significant blood loss, or that require skilled monitoring and nursing care post-procedure are generally not suitable for ambulatory patientspatients who will be admitted and discharged in the same day. However, note that ambulatory units associated with hospitals often accept and prepare patients for major and extensive surgery; these patients will be transferred to the appropriate postoperative unit after surgery. Also, some ambulatory units actually receive patients from the emergency room (such as a patient for an appendectomy or a woman with a miscarriage) to prepare for surgery. This demonstrates why the ambulatory nurse must maintain sharp skills.

### Support system

Ambulatory care means by definition that the patient will be out of the facility that same day. In this situation, someone must provide the aftercare that in a hospital would be performed by a trained nurse. So the ambulatory nurse must ascertain that the designated support person is indeed going to be able to provide that care. It is essential that the patient have adequate support care at home, and it is frequently the nurse who must determine if the support person will be able to meet these care requirements. When a patient arrives for ambulatory care without a support person who can demonstrate the ability to provide aftercare when indicated and take responsibility for the patient, the nurse should notify the physician of the situation. It may be necessary to reconsider accepting the patient as ambulatory. This is an area that will become more flexible as hospitals and other ambulatory facilities open special observation units and assisted care facilities for postprocedure care. Patients who are not ready to go home but who do not require the level of nursing care found in a hospital will appreciate this alternative.

### Third-party payer

As mentioned before, the third-party payer often makes the final decision on which patients will be treated as ambulatory and which will be hospitalized. When the physician, nurse, or anesthetist believe the patient is not suitable for ambulatory care and should be treated as an inpatient, it is up to them to act as patient advocates. This will no doubt be an area of heated debate as new health care reform measures are implemented.

### Physicians

Physicians have a tremendous influence on whether a patient will be treated as ambulatory or inpatient. Most patients follow their doctor's recommendation regarding hospitalization or ambulatory care. Physicians are influenced in that choice by their prior experience with ambulatory care, the patient's condition and preference, the ease and convenience of care, the type of procedure being considered, and their own schedules.

# NURSING CONSIDERATIONS

While nurses seldom make the final decision about inpatient versus ambulatory care, they can wield significant influence on that process. Below are listed a few ways that nurses can influence the selection of patients for ambulatory versus inpatient care.

- Join professional organizations of ambulatory care providers and form networking groups within your professional community. These groups may be formed by nurses from the ambulatory unit as well as perioperative and post-anesthesia nurses. Participation in professional groups gives you an opportunity to stay abreast of issues and developments in ambulatory patient care. There is strength in numbers; when united, nurses may influence third-party payers and others.

- Educate patients and community members about the benefits and drawbacks of ambulatory care. Nurses have always focused on returning patients to their highest level of wellness as soon as possible; ambulatory care exemplifies that goal.

- Never underestimate your power as a nurse; neither surgeons nor insurers will get much work done without a nurse.

- Act as patient advocate when a patient cannot demonstrate the support essential to safe home aftercare. Discharging a patient with inadequate support or aftercare arrangements is ethically unsound and may leave the staff and facility open to legal liability.

## SUMMARY

This chapter described how patients are selected for ambulatory care and the types of procedures most amenable to the ambulatory setting. Patient selection based on age, health status, nature of the procedure, support system, physician, and third-party payers was reviewed. While ambulatory patients ideally are in good health with a strong support system, the reality is that more complex procedures are being performed on sicker patients. The final determination on ambulatory versus inpatient care is often made by a third-party payer. Ambulatory nurses must be prepared to meet this challenge and act as patient advocates when necessary. Considerations for the ambulatory patient care nurse were also presented.

## CRITICAL CONCEPTS

- Factors influencing the decision to provide ambulatory care versus inpatient care include: patient age and health status, the nature of the procedure, the availability of adequate support for aftercare, third-party payers, and the patient's physician.

- Patients most suitable for ambulatory care (admission and discharge in the same day) include those who are healthy or have a well controlled mild chronic disease process, are undergoing procedures involving approximately 4 hours or less of general anesthesia (when administered) and do not have a high incidence of complication or major blood loss, and those who will not require extensive skilled nursing care postoperatively.

- Nurses can influence the evolution of ambulatory care by staying abreast of developments in the field and by forming or joining professional organizations in the field of ambulatory care.

- Third-party payers often will make the final decision as to whether a patient will be treated as ambulatory or inpatient.

- The patient should have adequate support at home for care after an ambulatory procedure.

# EXAM QUESTIONS

## Chapter 4

Questions 11-13

11. The final decision as to whether a patient will be treated as ambulatory versus inpatient often rests with the:

    a. patient
    b. third-party payer
    c. family
    d. anesthetist

12. For which one of these procedures would the patient likely be hospitalized?

    a. D&C
    b. cystoscopy
    c. tonsillectomy
    d. pneumonectomy

13. Referring to the American Society of Anesthesiologists Physical Status (PS) Classifications, which classes of patients are most suitable for ambulatory surgery?

    a. PS 4 & PS 5
    b. PS 1, PS 3, PS 4
    c. PS 1 & PS 2
    d. PS 4 & PS 6E

# CHAPTER 5

# CONSIDERATIONS IN AMBULATORY ANESTHESIA: GENERAL ANESTHESIA

## CHAPTER OBJECTIVE

After reading this chapter, you should be able to define general anesthesia, recognize fundamental aspects of the administration of general anesthesia, specify the pharmacologic agents commonly used in the ambulatory setting, and then based on this knowledge, plan nursing care for the ambulatory patient undergoing general anesthesia.

## LEARNING OBJECTIVES

After reading this chapter, you should be able to:

1. Recognize the definition of general anesthesia.

2. Identify inhalation and intravenous agents commonly used in ambulatory anesthesia and their impact on nursing care.

3. Specify common nursing diagnoses for the patient undergoing general anesthesia.

4. Choose nursing actions that enhance the safety and comfort of the ambulatory patient undergoing general anesthesia.

5. Recognize fundamental aspects of the administration of general anesthesia.

6. Identify monitors commonly used during general anesthesia.

## INTRODUCTION

Advances in anesthesia have been a major factor in the current widespread trend towards ambulatory surgery. New pharmacologic anesthetic agents reduce recovery time and make it possible for patients to be "street-ready" much sooner than ever before. These new agents and the subsequent advances in ambulatory anesthesia make anesthesia quite safe for most patients. Nevertheless, for many patients, "going under" anesthesia remains one of the most frightening aspects of ambulatory surgery. Because fear and anxiety can stimulate the sympathetic nervous system, the nurse who can allay a patient's fears, once again, has an opportunity to positively influence the outcome of the procedure. Armed with a basic knowledge of the fundamentals of anesthesia, the ambulatory nurse who prepares patients for surgery will be able to respond to many of the patient's concerns. This is not intended to suggest that the nurse should take on the responsibility of addressing all of the patient's concerns about anesthesia; that is the responsibility of the anesthesia provider. But knowledge is power, and an understanding of the basic facts about anesthesia can enhance the nurse's care of the ambulatory patient undergoing general anesthesia.

This chapter reviews those basic fundamental aspects of general anesthesia and describes common pharmacologic agents used in that process, with the emphasis on those agents that are most commonly used in ambulatory anesthesia. Written to enhance your understanding of general anesthesia, this chapter also includes strategies for the nurse caring for the ambulatory patient undergoing general anesthesia; it closes with a summary of the material presented and a list of the critical concepts.

# GENERAL ANESTHESIA

Anesthesia means loss of sensation. A state of altered physiology characterized by unconsciousness and insensibility to pain, general anesthesia (GA) is administered for the purpose of allowing surgery or other painful procedures to be completedprocedures that would otherwise be impossible because of the pain involved (or in some cases because the patient would be unable to cooperate, as in pediatrics). Modern anesthesia generally makes surgery safer and certainly more humane.

Surgery causes pain. Pain stimulates the sympathetic nervous system and thereby triggers the "fight or flight" mechanism; the result is an increase in heart rate and blood pressure. Unchecked, this response could lead to a hypertensive crisis, stroke, cardiac arrhythmias, cardiac arrest, and even death. GA blunts this stress response to the pain of surgical manipulation. In addition to the obvious benefit of rendering the patient unconscious and therefore unaware of the pain of surgery, anesthesia also helps reduce this sympathetic response to the pain of surgical stimulation.

General anesthesia does more than produce unconsciousness and unawareness of the surgery; it also has other effects that are usually desirable, depending upon the type of surgery. General anesthesia is characterized by amnesia (lack of recall), by analgesia (relief from pain), and by muscle relaxation. These three effects, amnesia, analgesia, and muscle relaxation, are referred to as the triad of general anesthesia. Each component takes on varying degrees of importance based upon the type of surgery being performed.

General anesthesia is usually administered as a combination of drugs and anesthetic agents that are injected intravenously (IV) and inhaled. However, advances in the development of anesthetic agents have made possible total intravenous anesthesia (TIVA), a technique that is especially amenable to the ambulatory care setting. In this case, no inhaled anesthetic agents are administered (although the gases oxygen and nitrous oxide are included as part of the anesthetic). General anesthesia is also sometimes administered solely with an inhalation agent, without the use of IV agents. This anesthetic technique is usually restricted to brief pediatric procedures. The process of administering GA encompasses three phases: induction, maintenance, and recovery, which are discussed below.

## Induction

In the first half of this century, before intravenous (IV) induction agents were widely used, general anesthesia was induced by having the patient inhale an anesthetic agent such as ether. This is an inhalation induction. As the patient inhaled, consciousness was gradually lost. Unfortunately, the patient passed through several phases including, excitement, that involved some coughing and struggling, before the plane of surgical anesthesia (a level of anesthesia where the patient does not react to the pain of incision) was reached. These phases could result in difficulty managing the patient's airway, so inhalation inductions are seldom utilized now, except in young children who cannot cooperate with insertion of an intravenous cannula. Modern anesthetists use IV hypnotic agents such as sodium thiopental (Pentothal) or propofol (Diprivan) to bypass these unpleasant stages, rapidly induce unconsciousness, and advance directly to a plane of surgical anesthesia. This is called an intravenous induction; it induces unconsciousness in the patient. After induction of anesthesia the patient's airway is secured either by the use of an oral or nasal airway or an endotracheal tube. This allows the anesthetist to insure the flow of oxygen to the patient's lungs. During administration of the anesthetic the anesthetist may completely control the patient's respirations, assist the patent's own efforts to breathe, or allow the patient to breathe spontaneously. Securing a patent airway is an obviously essential task of every anesthetic, and surgery should not proceed until this is accomplished.

## Maintenance

Because most induction agents are so short acting, GA must be maintained by the continued administration of anesthetic agents and other drugs that are adjuncts to anesthesia. Often the patient breathes in an inhalation anesthetic agent. This is delivered from the anesthesia machine to the patient via an anesthesia mask or endotracheal tube. In some cases, especially short operations, IV agents may be used to maintain general anesthesia without the addition of inhalation agents. Such is the case with TIVA, which is an increasingly popular technique, especially in ambulatory surgery.

Based on the patient's response to the surgery, the depth of the anesthetic is altered by increasing or decreasing the amount of anesthetic agents delivered to the patient. It is interesting to note that even though the patient may be rendered unconscious by the anesthetic agent, the sympathetic nervous system's "fight or flight" mechanism can still be stimulated by the pain of surgical manipulation. This response usually is heralded by an increase in the heart rate and blood pressure, and it may precipitate a hypertensive crisis, cardiac arrhythmias stimulated by catecholamine (stress hormones) release, tearing of the eyes, and even movement by the patient. In this case, the anesthetic depth is considered to be too "light," and more anesthetic agents are administered to allow the surgery to proceed safely. On the opposite end of the spectrum, the sympathetic nervous system can be profoundly depressed by the anesthetic level. In this case, the blood pressure may fall dangerously low and the heart may stop. At this point, the patient is said to be too "deep." The challenge for the anesthetist is to balance the patient between these two extremes. In some patients, such as the elderly, those with cardiovascular disease, and trauma victims, this can be difficult and may require constant adaptation and response on the part of the anesthetist.

## Emergence

As the procedure nears completion, the anesthetist gradually reduces the amounts of anesthetic delivered to the patient and the patient begins awakening. General anesthesia is not simply undone when the administration of anesthetic agents and the surgery stop; it is a process that may take several hours and is marked by the gradual return of reflexes and patient awakening. Since the patient is still under the influence of some of the anesthetic agents until recovery is complete, he or she must be monitored carefully, preferably by a specially trained nurse who has expertise and skills in this specialty. Sometimes it is necessary to reverse with other drugs (reversal agents) the effects of the drugs administered for the anesthetic.

## Special considerations in general anesthesia for the ambulatory patient

Administration of general anesthesia to the ambulatory patient involves a number of concerns. Ideally, recovery from general anesthesia is prompt with minimal side effects such as drowsiness, dizziness, or nausea and vomiting. If complications do arise, it is preferable that these complications develop while the patient is still in the facility and can receive professional intervention, rather than after discharge. Prompt recovery from anesthesia is especially desirable in ambulatory settings for several reasons. First, patients who are street-ready sooner mean a faster turnover of beds and more efficient utilization of the facility and personnel. Since efficient utilization of health care facilities is most certainly going to be increasingly emphasized in the future, this is a challenging arena for change. Second, ambulatory patients are generally eager to return to the comfort of their homes to recuperate. Third, prompt recovery from the effects of anesthesia boosts confidence that anesthetic complications most likely are not going to occur after the patient is discharged.

## Indications for general anesthesia

General anesthesia is administered for the purpose of allowing surgery or other uncomfortable procedures to proceed without pain. Inducing anesthesia, or loss of sensation, in just the area of the body where the surgery will be performed certainly makes sense, especially in ambulatory settings. However, even though many procedures can be adequately or even more safely performed under local anesthesia or with a regional anesthetic technique, the majority of patients usually prefer GA because they are frightened of being awake during their operation. Many surgeons and anesthetists also prefer general anesthesia because it is usually rapidly induced and reliable in effect. The same cannot always be said for regional or local anesthetic techniques, a topic that will be discussed in the following chapter. Aside from patient and professional preference, there are some other factors that must be considered when choosing an anesthetic technique.

- **Patient age and mental status:** Children, some elderly patients, and others who lack the necessary mobility and mental acuity to cooperate often require GA rather than regional or local anesthesia.

- **Type of surgery:** Regional anesthetic techniques are generally (but not always) limited in duration by time, so an operation that is expected to take longer than the appropriate regional anesthetic can be expected to endure is usually performed under general anesthesia. Also, some surgical procedures may require patient positioning or use of surgical instruments that the conscious patient would simply find too uncomfortable. In these cases, GA is usually chosen.

## Contraindications to general anesthesia

There are few absolute contraindications to general anesthesia when the proposed surgery is considered essential or even life saving. However, most ambulatory surgeries do not fall into this category. Since many ambulatory procedures are elective and the patient is expected to leave the facility that day, patients should be screened carefully before selection as ambulatory candidates for general anesthesia.

- **Full stomach:** Patients are generally asked to have nothing by mouth, including liquids and solids, for at least 6 hours before GA is to be administered; many anesthetists consider GA contraindicated if the patient has not adhered to this fasting order. This is because under certain conditions anything in the patient's stomach could flow back up into the esophagus and then be inhaled into the lungs during GA. The regurgitation can be passive (reflux) or active (vomiting). This mishap can cause a fatal aspiration pneumonitis; only a small amount (cc) of aspirated gastric secretions can result in death (Roberts & Shirley, 1976). However, recent research challenges the long-standing assumption that fasting reduces the risk of aspiration (Maltby, et al, 1986). For now, most authorities still consider fasting before general anesthesia essential in the struggle to prevent aspiration; nurses should watch for future developments on fasting requirements and consult their own institution's policy guidelines. More information about aspiration can be found in Chapter 14.

- **Abnormal preanesthesia tests:** In most cases, the patient's hematocrit should be at least 30% for elective surgery. Other blood and urine studies, chest x-ray, and electrocardiogram (ECG) should ideally be within normal limits before GA is administered to the ambulatory patient. Unfortunately, this is not always possible, due to the fact that patients who are less than healthy are being channeled into the ambulatory care system. The decision to proceed with general anesthesia and surgery, in the face of abnormal test results and complicated medical conditions, rests with the surgeon, the anesthetist, and the patient, and is influenced by a number of factors, including the insurer.

- **Medical disease:** When first developed, ambulatory care was targeted at healthy patients; those with medical illnesses were referred for inpatient care. However, health care cost containment measures now dictate that not only well, but often quite ill, patients will be treated on an ambulatory basis; these decisions may be made by the patient's insurer. The staff at the ambulatory facility will have to take the patient's status into account when determining whether or not to accept the patient for the ambulatory procedure.

# INTRAVENOUS AGENTS USED DURING ANESTHESIA

As mentioned before, pharmacologic advances in anesthesia have been a significant factor in the increased utilization of ambulatory surgery. These advances have resulted in drugs and anesthetic agents that are short acting and more easily controlled during the anesthetic. The short duration of action is not only ideal for shorter ambulatory procedures, but the short duration also means that the patient will generally awaken sooner even when the drug is used for a longer procedure. Many of these newer agents also help enhance the safety of anesthesia because of a lower incidence of undesirable effects.

Table 5-1 lists common intravenous agents used in general anesthesia; these agents are reviewed in the following sections. Professionals who administer these drugs must have advanced training in skills in managing the effects of these drugs. The information about these drugs is presented solely to enhance your understanding of anesthesia. It is neither a guide to nor a recommendation for your administration of any of these drugs or agents.

## Narcotics

Narcotics are opioid analgesics; they act on the opioid receptors in the brain. Opioid analgesics relieve pain, sedate, and blunt the sympathetic "fight or flight" stress response to surgery and endotracheal intubation. Narcotics can also reduce blood pressure and slow the heart rate in the perioperative period. For these reasons, most ambulatory patients having surgery under general anesthesia will receive an IV dose of a narcotic just before or during induction. While narcotics do induce drowsiness and can theoretically delay discharge of the ambulatory patient, eliminating their use in all but brief and relatively non-painful procedures is generally not helpful. This is because the patient who received no narcotic before or during surgery will usually complain of pain upon awakening from anesthesia, and will subsequently have to be medicated then, thus delaying discharge.

Sometimes narcotics are used as the primary anesthetic agent in a technique known as narcotic anes-

## Table 5-1
## Common Intravenous Anesthesia Agents

| Drug Classification | Use in anesthesia | Examples (during anesthesia, these drugs are commonly administered IV by the anesthetist) |
|---|---|---|
| Tranquilizers | Allay anxiety, sedation | Benzodiazepines: midazolam (Versed), diazepam (Valium), lorazepam (Ativan). The first reversal agent for benzodiazepines, flumazenil (Romazicon), was introduced in 1992. |
| | Antinauseant, sedation | Butyrophenone: droperidol (Inapsine) <br> Phenothiazine: promethazine (Phenergan) |
| Narcotics | Analgesia, sedation, blunt sympathetic response to surgical stimulation | Fentanyl (Sublimaze), Sufentanil (Sufenta), Alfentanil (Alfenta). The action of narcotics can be reversed with the narcotic antagonist naloxone (Narcan). |
| Agonist-antagonists | Analgesia, sedation | Butorphanol (Stadol), Nalbuphine (Nubain). These drugs generally produce less respiratory depression than pure opioid agonists such as fentanyl or morphine and can be used to reverse some of the effects of narcotics. |
| Non-narcotic, non-barbiturate hypnotic agents | Sedation, hypnosis, induction of anesthesia | Etomidate (Amidate); Propofol (Diprivan) also used for maintenance of general anesthesia (TIVA). Induces sedation or unconsciousness in a dose-dependent fashion. |
| Barbiturates | Sedation, hypnosis, induction of anesthesia | Sodium pentothal (Thiopental), thiamylal (Surital), methohexital (Brevital). May be for sedation or to induce unconsciousness, depending on dosage. |
| Dissociative agent | Analgesia, induction (and sometimes maintenance) of anesthesia | Ketamine (Ketalar). More often used in children; may be the sole anesthetic agent for some short procedures. |
| Neuromuscular blocking agents | Facilitate intubation, provide muscle relaxation for surgical procedure or for manipulation | Depolarizing: Succinylcholine (Quelicin, Anectine) <br> Non-depolarizing: Pancuronium (Pavulon), atracurium (Tracrium), vecuronium (Norcuron), pipecuronium (Arduan), mivacurium (Mivacron), doxacurium (Nuromax), curare. |

thesia. In this case, higher doses of narcotics are given IV to provide analgesia; nitrous oxide ("laughing gas") and oxygen are administered to produce amnesia; a neuromuscular blocking drug that produces muscle relaxation is injected IV, and this completes the triad of anesthesia. However, this technique is not as popular in ambulatory anesthesia because the patient is often quite drowsy after longer procedures with higher doses of narcotics. More commonly in ambulatory settings, small doses of narcotics such as fentanyl (Sublimaze) or alfentanil (Alfenta) are used along with other anesthetic agents. The nurse should note that the effects of narcotics can be reversed by the administration of naloxone (Narcan), but this often results in the acute awareness of pain and may necessitate re-medicating the patient for this pain.

In summary, narcotics are used in anesthesia for analgesia, sedation, and to blunt the body's stress response to surgery and endotracheal intubation. The effects of narcotics can generally be reversed by naloxone (Narcan).

## Tranquilizers

Tranquilizers are integrated into the anesthesia care plan for the purpose of sedating the patient and allaying anxiety (anxiolysis), and for reducing recall (amnesia) of perioperative events, an effect many patients find desirable. Recent pharmacologic advances have produced a tranquilizer that is short acting and as such is especially suited to the ambulatory setting: midazolam (Versed). This benzodiazepine tranquilizer is water soluble, thereby causing less pain upon injection than its precursor diazepam (Valium). While diazepam was known for its long duration of action and its "second peak" effect that could release active metabolites hours after administration, midazolam has found widespread acceptance in ambulatory procedures because of its properties. However, midazolam (Versed) is two to four times more potent that diazepam (Valium) (White, et al, 1988) so overdosages have been fatal. This drug must be carefully titrated to the patient's response and condition. In 1992, the first reversal agent for benzodiazepines, flumazenil (Romazicon), was introduced. This drug should prove to be a breakthrough in ambulatory anesthesia, because it can reverse or attentuate the effects of benzodiazepines just as naloxone (Narcan) reverses the effects of narcotics.

Some tranquilizers the (butyrophenones and the phenothiazines) also reduce or eliminate nausea. The butyrophenone droperidol (Inaspine), which belongs to the same class of drugs as haloperidol (Haldol), a major tranquilizer, enjoys widespread popularity in ambulatory anesthesia because of its antinauseant properties. Generally, only small doses (0.625 1.25 mg or even less) are necessary to achieve this effect. Larger doses of droperidol can cause unpleasant psychic effects and are generally avoided when this drug is used for its antinauseant effect.

In summary, tranquilizers are used in anesthesia to sedate the patient, reduce anxiety, limit recall or induce amnesia (benzodiazepines), and as antinauseants (phenothiazines and butyrophenones). A reversal agent for the benzodiazepines, flumazenil (Romazicon) was recently introduced into clinical practice.

## Agonist-antagonist agents

The agonist-antagonist drugs such as nalbuphine (Nubain) and butorphanol (Stadol) act on opioid receptors in the brain. In the patient who has received an opioid analgesic, these drugs in small doses can maintain that analgesia while reversing some of the depressant effects of the opioid. Respiratory depression after administration of an agonist-antagonist agent is generally less than that with opioid analgesics, so these drugs are often used in the absence of narcotics and seem to be enjoying an increase in use in some ambulatory settings. In the narcotic-addicted patient, the nurse should note that agonist-antagonists can precipitate an acute withdrawal response.

In summary, the agonist-antagonist agents are used in anesthesia to provide sedation and analgesia, and may be used in certain circumstances to reverse the respiratory depressant effects of opioid analgesics, or narcotics. The effects of agonist-antagonist agents can generally be reversed by naloxone (Narcan).

## Non-narcotic, non-barbiturate hypnotic agents

Hypnotic agents are those that induce sleep or loss of consciousness. There are currently two hypnotics that belong to neither the narcotic nor the barbiturate families: propofol (Diprivan) and etomidate (Amidate). Propofol has revolutionized the practice of ambulatory anesthesia since its introduction in 1990. A milky-looking white emulsion, propofol is popular in ambulatory anesthesia because the patient's recovery is usually swift, as validated by the return of reflexes and psychomotor skills. The level of patient alertness after the administration of propofol is often extraordinary compared to other hypnotic agents. Propofol doesn't leave patients quite as groggy or with a "hung over" feeling. Propofol is injected IV to induce and/or maintain anesthesia according to a dose-dependent effect, and is often a major component of a TIVA technique for the ambulatory surgery patient. In this case, a syringe of propofol is usually connected to a pump that delivers the drug to the patient's IV tubing; the amount is titrated to the patient's response. Consciousness is lost about 60 seconds after a bolus dose of the drug. Nausea is generally less after propofol than after a barbiturate, but this drug does sometimes cause pain upon IV injection. Propofol also depresses the cardiovascular system and may result in hypotension. Due to the nature of the emulsion, propofol can support microbial growth; it must be discarded if not used within six hours. Etomidate (Amidate) is not as widely used as propofol or the barbiturates in anesthesia.

In summary, non-narcotic, non-barbiturate hypnotic agents are used in anesthesia for sedation or induction of anesthesia, which is loss of consciousness. Propofol may also be used to maintain anesthesia for surgery. There is no reversal agent for either of these drugs, but the short duration of action does not make this a drawback.

## Barbiturates

Most nurses are familiar with the family of barbiturates that include such drugs as secobarbital (Seconal) which is sometimes ordered for sleep. From within this class of drugs come the ultra-short acting barbiturates that are used intravenously in anesthesia. Since their introduction over 50 years ago, barbiturates such as sodium pentothal (Thiopental) have been the most common anesthetic induction agents. These ultra-short acting barbiturates can be injected IV in low doses to sedate the patient or in higher doses to induce unconsciousness. Patients lose consciousness about 20 seconds after injection of a bolus dose; some note a garlic-like taste in the mouth at this time. Because these drugs can cause histamine release, a red rash is occasionally noted across the patient's chest. Sometimes associated with nausea and vomiting, the barbiturates have a duration of action longer than propofol, and the patient's return to preanesthesia level of functioning is not as rapid.

In summary, ultra-short acting barbiturates are used in anesthesia to produce sedation or induce unconsciousness. There is no reversal agent for barbiturates.

## Dissociative agent

Administered IV or IM, ketamine (Ketalar) produces unconsciousness and profound analgesia. A phencyclidine similar to the illicit drug PCP, ketamine has been associated with emergence delirium, hallucinations, and psychic side effects ranging from unpleasant to serious. Ketamine functionally dissociates parts of the brain, so the patient does not react to pain. Although he or she may appear to be awake during the procedure, the patient receiving ketamine will seldom have any recall of the event. Ketamine also stimulates the cardiovascular system and therefore supports the blood pressure. Because the respirations generally remain strong and it can be injected IM, ketamine may be used outside of the Operating Rooms in other anesthetizing locations (such as radiology), or even outside of the hospital itself in certain emergency or disaster situations. One of the most common uses of ketamine in ambulatory anesthesia is in children, such as those undergoing cardiac catheterization. A major drawback of ketamine is the high incidence of postoperative hallucinations, although these can be reduced by the concurrent administration of diazepam (Valium) and providing a quiet, non-stimulating environment (skillful neglect).

In summary, ketamine is used to provide analgesia and induce anesthesia. It is not widely used in ambulatory adult patients; it is more commonly used in pediatrics. There is no reversal agent for ketamine.

### Neuromuscular blocking agents

Nurses will hear the neuromuscular blocking agents referred to casually in surgery as "muscle relaxants," but it is essential to note that these drugs bear no similarity to muscle relaxants prescribed for ailments such as back strains. These neuromuscular blocking agents prevent the transfer of impulses across the neuromuscular junction, which is the microscopic area where nerves attach to skeletal muscles. With this junction blocked, the nerve impulses do not reach, or are impeded in reaching, the muscle. The result is that the muscles become weak or unable to respond, effectively paralyzing the patient. There are two types of neuromuscular blocking agents: depolarizing and nondepolarizing. An example of a depolarizing agent is succinylcholine (Anectine); nondepolarizing agents include pancuronium (Pavulon) or vecuronium (Norcuron).

Neuromuscular blocking agents are administered during anesthesia (and sometimes in a hospital's critical care areas) to provide the third component of the triad of anesthesia, which is muscle relaxation. This muscle relaxation facilitates exposure of internal organs and allows placement of surgical instruments such as retractors. This is accomplished by the relaxing of the abdominal or chest muscles that results from the action of the neuromuscular blocking agent. Muscle relaxation is also employed in certain orthopedic procedures to allow easier manipulation of the joint, and is an essential part of GA when any chance of patient movement is undesirable, as in ophthalmic surgery. Because the patient's muscles are weakened or paralyzed by these drugs, the patient's respirations must be supported. That is why these drugs should be administered only by those trained to manage the airway and ventilate the patient, because respiratory efforts will usually cease or become ineffective after administration. Airway management equipment must be immediately available when these drugs are injected. Note that these drugs have no effect on mentation or pain: neuromuscular blocking agents do not provide analgesia or amnesia. They simply paralyze the muscles, and while the patient may appear unconscious, this is not the case unless narcotics, tranquilizers, or other anesthetic agents are administered concurrently. This can have important implications for the staff and the patient, because the patient may be aware of conversations and may feel intense pain, but will be unable to respond.

The action of the non-depolarizing neuromuscular blocking agents is usually reversed at the completion of surgery by the administration of anticholinesterase agents such as neostigmine. An adequate dose of neostigmine will allow resumption of neuromuscular transmission and the patient's muscle tone, strength, and respirations should return. The anticholinesterase agents are usually administered concurrently with an anticholinergic, such as atropine, which will counteract some of the undesirable effects of the anticholinesterase agent. If reversal of the neuromuscular blocking agent is not complete or feasible, the patient will require ventilatory support until the effects of the agent wear off.

In summary, neuromuscular blocking agents are drugs used to paralyze the patient or reduce muscle tone during surgery. These potent drugs will also halt or render ineffective the patient's attempts at breathing, so the respirations must be supported. The nondepolarizing drugs are usually reversed by an anticholinesterase after surgery.

# INHALATION AGENTS USED IN GENERAL ANESTHESIA

After induction, general anesthesia must be maintained for the duration of the procedure. While intravenous agents are sometimes used to maintain anesthesia (as in TIVA), maintenance is usually accomplished by the administration of an inhalation anesthetic agent.

### Inhalation anesthetic agents

These agents are supplied as liquids which are heated to the vapor stage by the anesthesia machine, and then delivered to the patient in a carrier gas such as oxygen. The patient inhales this mixture, the blood in the lungs picks up the inhalation agent, and it is transported to the brain where it induces unconsciousness. There are currently four inhalation anesthetics in common use in the United States: halothane (Fluothane), enflurane (Ethrane), isoflurane (Forane), and desflurane (Suprane). Halothane is a halogenated hydrocarbon, but the other agents are halogenated ethers. These are derived from one of the first inhalation anesthetic agents, ether, which is no longer in use.

- **Halothane (Fluothane):** Most commonly used for inhalation inductions in children, halothane has a sweet smell and is not as irritating to the airway as the other agents which are derived from ether. Halothane does sensitize the heart to catecholamine (stress hormone) release, and serious or fatal arrhythmias can result, especially if the surgeon is also injecting epinephrine during the course of the procedure. Halothane at one time was questionably linked with some cases of postoperative hepatitis and so is usually not administered to patients with a history of liver disorders. Halothane is also a bronchodilator and as such is sometimes considered useful in asthmatic patients. The principal use of halothane today seems to be as an inhalation agent for children.

- **Enflurane (Ethrane):** Enflurane enjoyed wider use before the introduction of isoflurane in the '80s and desflurane in the '90s. It is still used for maintenance of anesthesia and is generally regarded as safe. There has been some controversy that enflurane might be linked with renal failure and seizures, so it is usually avoided in patients susceptible to these problems.

- **Isoflurane (Forane):** Isoflurane is one of the most popular inhalation anesthetic agents because it is mostly excreted by the lungs; only a tiny amount is metabolized by the body and excreted by the kidneys. This is an excellent benefit in the patient with impaired metabolic functions. And because it is excreted largely unchanged, most authorities believe patients can undergo multiple anesthetics with isoflurane without any cumulative toxic effects. This is often a source of comfort to patients who have multiple anesthetics and are concerned about cumulative effects on their bodies.

- **Desflurane (Suprane):** Only recently introduced, desflurane represents a significant advance in ambulatory anesthesia because of its short duration of action; rapid patient awakening occurs after administration ceases. This effect means that patients will arouse sooner and be more alert; this is an obvious advantage in ambulatory care.

## Carrier gases

As mentioned above, the inhalation agents are delivered to the patient's lungs via a carrier gas such as oxygen. Note that oxygen and nitrous oxide are actually gases, whereas the inhalation anesthetic agents described above are liquids that are heated to a vapor state for delivery to the patient's lungs. The three carrier gases commonly used in anesthesia are described below. Even when a TIVA technique is used without an inhalation anesthetic agent, oxygen and nitrous oxide are still employed.

- **Oxygen:** Oxygen must always be administered during GA to prevent the development of hypoxia. The concentration of oxygen delivered to the patient may range from 100% (the maximum) to little more than the oxygen content of room air, which is 21%. The amount chosen for delivery to the patient is determined by the anesthetist and is based on the type of anesthetic, the type of surgical procedure, and the patient's condition.

- **Nitrous oxide:** Nitrous oxide is also known as "laughing gas" and is used in anesthesia to produce amnesia and analgesia. It is commonly mixed with the oxygen for delivery to the patient. In certain patients and surgical procedures, nitrous oxide is contraindicated or undesirable.

- **Air:** Many modern anesthesia machines now provide air that can be mixed with the oxygen that is delivered to the patient. This allows a reduction in the amount of oxygen inspired by the patient; this can be valuable in the patient with chronic lung disease.

# MONITORING IN ANESTHESIA

Patient monitoring in anesthesia has come a long way from the "finger on the pulse" technique used a century ago. The standards of care for monitoring the patient receiving anesthesia are still evolving; this is an area that will experience dynamic changes in the future as computers are increasingly utilized in anesthesia care. It is important to know however that despite the wealth of monitors available during general anesthesia, the anesthetist remains the primary monitor of the patient.

Nurses can reassure ambulatory patients that they should receive the same level of monitoring during anesthesia that inpatients receive; just because the anesthetic is administered in a physician's office or freestanding clinic does not lower the standard of monitoring expected. Because some patients believe the anesthetist leaves after inducing anesthesia, it may also be helpful to inform the patient that the anesthetist is expected to be continually present with the patient during the anesthetic. Monitors often used in GA are briefly reviewed below. Knowing the types of monitoring used in GA will give you confidence in answering questions your patient may have during preoperative teaching. Described below are the monitors most commonly used during GA:

- **Electrocardiogram:** A continuous display of the patient's heart rhythm.

- **End-tidal CO2:** The end-tidal $CO_2$ monitor samples the air leaving the patient's lungs; $CO_2$ is the waste product of metabolism and is excreted by the lungs. This monitor confirms the adequacy of ventilation and reveals other vital information, in addition to verifying correct placement of the endotracheal tube. The sampling port fits into the breathing circuit that is connected to the anesthesia machine.

- **Pulse oximeter:** The pulse oximeter assesses the amount of oxygen being carried by the red blood cells and thus reveals whether adequate amounts of oxygen are reaching the patient's tissue. The monitor does this by passing a wave of light through the tissue (usually via a painless probe attached to a finger, toe, or ear lobe). This data is displayed on the screen, and is often referred to by the health care professional as the "$O_2$ sat" or simply the "sat." The digital display reading is also accompanied by an audible tone that accompanies each heart beat and changes in pitch when the data changes. This non-invasive monitor yields such valuable information that it is widely used in many clinical areas, not just surgery.

- **Blood pressure:** The blood pressure is generally measured no less frequently than every five minutes during anesthesia, and often more frequently. An automatic electronic BP monitor is frequently used in anesthesia.

- **Heart and breath sounds:** Continuous auscultation of heart and breath sounds during anesthesia allows the anesthetist to react immediately to any change in these parameters. Most anesthetists have their own custom-made earpiece that connects to a stethoscope placed over the patient's precordium or to a slender tube that is slipped into the anesthetized patient's esophagus. This system allows the anesthetist to constantly monitor the patient's heart and breath sounds throughout the case, while keeping hands free to care for the patient.

- **Temperature:** Temperature is generally monitored in patients undergoing GA. Temperature may be assessed by liquid crystal skin temperature patches or electronically via skin or esophageal monitors.

- **Inspired oxygen:** Inspired oxygen is measured from the anesthesia breathing circuit by a monitor placed within that circuit. This monitor's alarm is triggered by concentrations that fall below the preset limit, often about 30%, so that if the oxygen source fails, the anesthetist will be alerted immediately. The inspired oxygen monitor assesses how much oxygen is delivered to the patient's lungs; a pulse oximeter assesses the amount of oxygen in the patient's bloodstream.

- **Nerve Stimulator:** The nerve stimulator is used to assess the degree of recovery from neuromuscular blocking agents. The monitor stimulates a nerve which will cause the muscle to contract if recovery is complete or in progress. Adequate recovery is essential for maintenance of respiratory function.

- **Others:** Other monitors used in GA include those that monitor the anesthesia equipment, such as ventilator and circuit pressure monitors. Other sophisticated monitors are under development.

# NURSING STRATEGIES FOR THE AMBULATORY PATIENT UNDERGOING GENERAL ANESTHESIA

It is not uncommon for surgical patients to be more anxious about anesthesia than they are about their surgery. This is because the concept of anesthesia is shrouded in myths and is poorly understood by the general public. For example, many patients worry they will reveal personal or intimate information when "going under." Armed with a basic knowledge of anesthesia, the nurse preparing the ambulatory patient for surgery can help debunk this misconception and others, thereby relieving the patient's anxiety. Preparing ambulatory patients for GA also

## Table 5-2
## Patient Monitors Commonly Used In General Anesthesia

| Monitor: | What It Does: |
| --- | --- |
| Electrocardiogram (ECG) | Continuously displays heart rhythm. |
| Blood Pressure (usually automated or electronic) | Measures blood pressure. |
| Pulse Oximeter | Assesses the amount of oxygen being carried to the patient's tissues; allows early detection of hypoxia. |
| Heart and Breath Sounds | Allows anesthetist to hear the ventilation of the lungs and assess the heart tones. |
| Temperature | Allows the anesthetist to monitor patient for changes in temperature that would require evaluation and/or treatment. |
| End-tidal $CO_2$ | Verifies adequacy of ventilation and confirms correct placement of endotracheal tube, among other functions. |
| Inspired Oxygen | Measures amount of oxygen being delivered to the patient from the anesthesia machine via the breathing circuit. |
| Nerve Stimulator | Stimulates nerve over muscle to evaluate the return of neuromuscular function after neuromuscular blocking agents have been administered. |

incurs the additional challenge of a limited amount of time in which to accomplish this mission. The ambulatory nurse's strategy is generally one of allowing the patient to express fears, addressing those concerns by providing information or asking the anesthetist to address them, and then offering support and comfort. Table 5-2 lists common nursing diagnoses for patients undergoing general anesthesia. Chapter 7 describes the actual preparation of the patient for the procedure and anesthesia; Chapter 8 describes nursing care of the patient during ambulatory procedures. The nursing strategies below are general actions you may take when caring for an ambulatory patient who is undergoing anesthesia. Your intervention should be within the scope of your institution's practice guidelines, consistent with your state's Nurse Practice Act, within the scope of your professional license, and commensurate with your skills and training.

General nursing actions you can take when an ambulatory patient requires general anesthesia include:

- Teach ambulatory patients that modern anesthetic agents, introduced in only the past few years, mean a quicker recovery from the effects

## Table 5-3
## Potential Nursing Diagnoses for Patients Undergoing General Anesthesia

| Nursing Diagnosis | Nursing intervention |
|---|---|
| Knowledge deficit related to lack of exposure (to GA) | Give clear concise explanations, using terminology appropriate to patient's level of understanding and reinforce often; answer patient's questions about anesthesia and ask the anesthetist to reinforce your teaching and/or address the patient's concerns; establish an atmosphere of trust that will not minimize importance of the patient's concerns; provide written information as appropriate. |
| Anxiety related to situational crisis (receiving GA) | Listen to patient and allow verbalization of concerns; offer verbal reassurance and gentle touch as indicated. Alter the environment when possible to reduce stress: reduce noise, provide privacy, minimize traffic through patient care area. |
| Fear, related to unfamiliarity (with GA) | Explore patient's fears, then address those issues or ask the anesthetist to answer these concerns. Common concerns are: fear of revealing personal information during anesthesia, fear of not waking up (death during anesthesia), fear of waking up during the procedure, and fear of intractable pain or vomiting postop. Reassure the patient as indicated and administer sedatives as ordered. |
| Coping related to personal vulnerability (during anesthesia) | Encourage patient to express concerns about "going under" anesthesia; answer questions and correct misconceptions; ask anesthetist to address patient's concerns about anesthesia. |

Please note this is a sample of potential nursing diagnoses and is not presented as, nor intended to be, a complete care plan for the ambulatory patient. More complete information can be found in a medical surgical nursing course and textbook.

Adapted from: *Nursing Diagnosis Reference Manual* by Sheila Sparks and Cynthia M. Taylor, Springhouse Corporation, 1991, and *Overview of Anesthesia* for Nurses by Linda Chitwood, Western Schools, 1992.

of the anesthetic and a reduction in the drowsy, groggy feeling many patients have experienced after surgery with older anesthetic agents. This should help reduce the patient's anxiety and increase the confidence of the support person who will monitoring the patient at home.

- Reassure the patient and support person that the professional staff will not send the patient home before criteria for discharge are met. This information can help reduce anxiety in the support person who may be concerned that the patient will be discharged before fully alert, or until pain or nausea is controlled.

- Tell the ambulatory patient that an antinauseant is commonly administered during general anesthesia and that modern anesthetic agents are associated with a much lower incidence of nausea and vomiting. While the patient cannot be guaranteed a nausea-free recovery, this information helps reduce the concern of many patients who have a history of nausea after general anesthesia. These patients and those who also suffer from motion sickness may benefit from the preoperative application of a transdermal scopolamine patch, which is discussed in Chapter 7.

- Acknowledge that the proposed procedure may result in pain but explain that analgesics are usually administered during general anesthesia to control this pain and that more can be administered upon awakening if the pain recurs. This helps reduce patient anxiety about pain management after the procedure.

- Respect the patient's fears about anesthesia even if trivial or misguided. Acknowledge those concerns and then correct misconceptions. Acknowledging the patient's concerns as legitimate helps boost the patient's confidence in the nurse. Belittling or ridiculing concerns expressed by the patient may damage the professional relationship and result in the delivery of less than optimal care.

- Explain to the patient who has undergone multiple anesthetics that the effects of anesthetics are not cumulative. This means that the patient in general does not need to worry about his or her body "getting too much anesthesia" after repeated surgeries.

- Tell adult patients that anesthesia is usually induced by an IV injection and takes only a matter of seconds. This helps relieve anxiety in patients who believe they will have to breathe ether through a mask for induction.

- Reassure patients that they do not reveal personal or confidential information during anesthesia, since this can relieve anxiety for certain patients.

- Tell patients that ether is no longer used in anesthesia because safer and more pleasant alternatives are available. This helps reduce anxiety in patients who may have had an unpleasant experience with ether anesthesia.

- Tell patients that the development of modern anesthetic agents and advanced monitoring techniques makes anesthesia safer than ever, although the patient should know that no one can guarantee the outcome of professional health care. Knowing that anesthesia is generally quite safe and that the staff will do their best to prevent mishaps relieves anxiety in most patients.

# SUMMARY

This chapter reviews fundamental aspects of general anesthesia and describes common pharmacologic agents used in that process, with the emphasis on those agents that are most commonly used in ambulatory anesthesia. This chapter was written to enhance the nurse's understanding of anesthesia so that he or she is better able to prepare ambulatory patients for general anesthesia. This chapter includes strategies for the nurse caring for the ambulatory patient undergoing general anesthesia; it closes with a summary of the material presented and a list of the critical concepts.

# CRITICAL CONCEPTS

- Anesthesia is commonly induced by IV hypnotic agents such as propofol (Diprivan) or a barbiturate such as sodium thiopental (Pentothal), but may be induced by inhalation of anesthetic agents, especially in children.

- Modern anesthesia agents make ambulatory surgery safer than ever, even for the patient who must have multiple surgical procedures. Awakening is much quicker and there is less drowsiness after administration of the newer anesthetic agents.

- Inhalation anesthetic agents are liquids that are heated to the vapor stage by the anesthesia machine and then delivered in a carrier gas such as oxygen to the patient's lungs via a breathing circuit.

- Neuromuscular blocking agents are commonly referred to as muscle relaxants, but these drugs paralyze or weaken the patient's muscles so that respirations may cease. These potent drugs must be administered only by professionals trained in their use and in airway management.

- The anesthetist is the primary monitor of the patient during anesthesia; the anesthetist does not leave the patient during anesthesia unless relieved by another competent anesthesia professional.

# EXAM QUESTIONS

## Chapter 5

Questions 14-23

14. The triad of general anesthesia includes:
    a. amnesia, analgesia, and unconsciousness
    b. amnesia, sedation, and muscle relaxation
    c. amnesia, analgesia, and paralysis
    d. amnesia, analgesia, and muscle relaxation *(circled)*

15. A new inhalation anesthetic agent popular in ambulatory anesthesia is:
    a. isoflurane (Forane)
    b. enfluranc (Ethrane)
    c. desfluranc (Suprane) *(circled)*
    d. hatothane (Fluothane)

16. A relatively new intravenous anesthetic agent that is increasingly popular in ambulatory anesthesia is:
    a. ketamine (Ketalar)
    b. thiamylal (Surital)
    c. diazepam (Valium)
    d. propofol (Diprivan) *(circled)*

17. A common fear patients share about general anesthesia is:
    a. paralysis
    b. revealing personal information *(circled)*
    c. losing bowel control
    d. separation anxiety

18. A monitor that assesses the amount of oxygen being carried to the patient's tissues is:
    a. electrocardiogram
    b. pulse oximeter *(circled)*
    c. blood pressure gauge
    d. end-tidal $CO_2$

19. The end-tidal $CO_2$ monitor placed in the anesthesia circuit verifies:
    a. correct placement of the endotracheal tube *(circled)*
    b. adequate oxygen in the lungs
    c. metabolic functioning of the cytoplasm
    d. cardiac arrhythmias

20. The three phases of general anesthesia are:
    a. awakening, arousal, and depression
    b. induction, emergence, and stimulation
    c. maintenance, arousal, and emergence
    d. induction, maintenance, and emergence *(circled)*

21. During anesthesia, the primary monitor of the patient is the:
    a. anesthetist *(circled)*
    b. pulse oximeter
    c. surgeon
    d. electrocardiogram

22. A common nursing diagnosis for the patient undergoing general anesthesia is:
    a. fear *(circled)*
    b. poisoning
    c. self-care deficit
    d. noncompliance

23. Drugs that paralyze the patient's muscles are:
    a. neuromuscular blocking agents *(circled)*
    b. curariform tranquilizers
    c. benzodiazepine relaxants
    d. inhalation agents

# CHAPTER 6

# CONSIDERATIONS IN AMBULATORY ANESTHESIA: REGIONAL ANESTHESIA, LOCAL ANESTHESIA, AND SEDATION

## CHAPTER OBJECTIVE

After reading this chapter, you should be better prepared to define regional and local anesthesia and conscious sedation, recognize the pharmacologic agents commonly used in these anesthetics, and be able to plan nursing care for the ambulatory patient undergoing one of these anesthetics.

## LEARNING OBJECTIVES

After reading this chapter, you should be able to:

1. Recognize the definition of regional anesthesia.

2. Recognize the definition of local anesthesia.

3. Recognize the definition of conscious sedation and monitored anesthesia care.

4. Discriminate among the different types of regional anesthesia.

5. Identify agents commonly used in regional and local anesthesia.

6. Specify common nursing diagnoses for the patient undergoing regional or local anesthesia or conscious sedation.

7. Choose nursing actions that enhance the safety and comfort of the ambulatory patient undergoing regional or local anesthesia or conscious sedation.

## INTRODUCTION

While general anesthesia remains the most popular type of anesthetic for the ambulatory surgical patient (Miller, 1990 p. 2033), regional and local anesthetic techniques hold an important place in ambulatory care. It is likely that these techniques will be increasingly utilized in the future as sicker patients come for ambulatory care. This chapter offers a basic overview of the fundamental aspects of regional and local anesthesia for the ambulatory patient. Different types of regional anesthesia are discussed; common indications, advantages, disadvantages, and complications of each are described. Conscious sedation, or monitored anesthesia care (MAC) is also reviewed. Common pharmacologic agents used in these anesthetics are briefly listed. General nursing strategies for the patient undergoing these anesthetics are described. The chapter closes with a summary of the material presented and a list of the critical concepts.

# REGIONAL ANESTHESIA

Anesthesia means loss of sensation; regional anesthesia (RA) refers to inducing this loss of sensation in a specific region or area of the body. Drugs known as local anesthetics (LA) are injected into a specific region of the body to induce this loss of sensation. While these techniques may be called by their specific name, such as spinal anesthesia, you will often hear a regional anesthetic technique called a "block." This is a reference to the effect of RA: the blocking of sensorimotor impulses to and from the brain. General anesthesia is popular among patients, surgeons, and anesthetists because it is rapid in onset, reliable in effect, and relatively easy to administer. Regional anesthesia requires special technical expertise and usually some additional time to administer, and is occasionally unreliable in effect. Nevertheless, RA is a logical choice for many ambulatory procedures because it anesthetizes only the area where the physician will be working and reduces the potential for somnolence and nausea postoperatively. Below you will find listed the general indications and contraindications of regional anesthesia.

## Indications

Indications for RA include surgery and the relief of chronic pain.

- Surgery: There is a RA technique for many surgical procedures. Factors to be considered when choosing RA for ambulatory procedures include the patient's preference and condition, the anesthetist's skill, the surgeon's skill and preference, and the surgery schedule.

- Pain management: Some RA techniques are administered in the ambulatory setting for the relief of chronic pain.

## Contraindications

RA is not appropriate for every ambulatory patient. Some of the more common contraindications to RA include:

- Coagulopathy: Patients on anticoagulants are seldom considered for RA because of the potential for bleeding around the puncture site where the LA is injected. This bleeding could compress nerves and might subsequently cause neuropathy.

- Patient preference: Even though RA may be the best choice for the patient and procedure, some patients will refuse due to misconceptions and fears about RA. Children and mentally impaired adults are seldom candidates for RA unless they are able to cooperate with placement.

- Medical disease: Certain disorders such as arthritis can make placement of a RA difficult because access to the site may be restricted by boney disease or impaired mobility of the patient. Septicemia and infection at the injection site precludes RA because of the risk of spreading the infection with needle insertion. Other conditions such as heart disease and anemia are relative contraindications to spinal anesthesia because some transient hypotension often develops with this technique and the body may be unable to compensate.

- Length of surgery: Regional anesthetic techniques generally are of fixed duration; if the surgery is expected to exceed this amount of time, RA may not be appropriate. An exception is when a catheter is placed (as in epidural anesthesia) so additional amounts of LA can be administered as needed.

# REGIONAL ANESTHESIA TECHNIQUES

Regional anesthesia refers to inducing loss of sensation in a specific region of the body. The most common types of RA used in the ambulatory setting include spinal, epidural, intravenous regional, and nerve blocks. These are described below, along with administration and the common indications, advantages, disadvantages, and complications of each. Note that intravenous access is secured before these techniques are attempted. This allows for the administration of intravenous (IV) agents as needed, and provides for the administration of emergency drugs should complications develop.

## Spinal anesthesia

Encircled by a sac of membranous tissue called the dura, the spinal cord carries sensations such as pain to the brain and transmits messages to our muscles so that we are mobile. The spinal cord ends around the second lumbar vertebrae in the lower back; it is bathed in cerebrospinal fluid (CSF). When a local anesthetic (LA) drug is injected into this fluid, the result is loss of sensation (anesthesia) from that point on down. This is called spinal anesthesia and is also referred to as a subarachnoid block (SAB). The actual puncture of the dura and injection of LA are made below the area where the spinal cord ends, so there is little risk of injury to the cord itself.

The amount of LA used, the area of injection, and the patient's position generally determine the resulting level of anesthesia. The patient experiences loss of sensation from the area that the LA affects on down. For example, if the LA spread up to the fourth thoracic vertebra, the patient would be numb from the nipples down. The LA interrupts impulses traveling to and from the brain, blocking perception of pain but also vasomotor control. As a result, the vessels dilate and the blood pressure may fall, although this is generally countered by a bolus of intravenous fluid before the anesthetic is administered.

- Administration: With the patient sitting or lying with the back arched (to help spread the vertebral interspaces), the area of administration (usually the second, third, or fourth lumbar interspace) is cleansed and draped. Using a sterile technique, the anesthetist inserts a fine gauge (usually 22-26 gauge) needle until CSF is noted at the hub of the needle, confirming proper placement. The LA is injected into the CSF and the patient is positioned for maximum effectiveness (the LA will begin acting immediately so the patient must be positioned quickly). For example, for a D & C the patient would most likely be kept sitting to prevent the rise of the LA in the CSF. This helps insure numbness only of the perineum and pelvic structures (this is called a "saddle block" because it numbs the areas that would touch a saddle) and prevents the development of a more extensive SAB. For intra-abdominal procedures, the patient immediately lies flat or even trendelenburg to help the anesthetic spread higher up the back, thus increasing the level of anesthesia.

- Indications: SAB is most often used for procedures on the lower body and lower extremities.

- Advantages: SAB is rapid in onset and generally reliable in inducing complete loss of sensation.

- Disadvantages: SAB is of limited duration, although at some facilities a catheter may be inserted for continuous LA administration to prolong the SAB. However, this may increase the chance of a spinal headache postoperatively.

- Potential complications: Because spinal anesthesia involves piercing the dura to inject LA, some CSF will inevitably be lost. This results in less CSF to cushion the brain in the skull, and the patient may develop a headache upon standing as the brain sinks down in the cranium. This spinal headache is relieved by recumbency. To prevent this, some anesthetists require patients to lie flat for 12 to 24 hours after a spinal anesthetic–an obvious disadvantage in ambulatory care. However, experts are now debating whether this restriction is necessary. Increasing fluid intake may also help replenish the CSF. Because the incidence of spinal headache is significantly reduced in patients over 60, many clinicians restrict spinal anesthesia in ambulatory settings to those past this age. Another potential complication is hypotension, which can be profound as vasomotor control is lost; patients with cardiovascular disease may be unable to compensate. Also, the level of SAB can rise higher than intended, causing the patient to stop breathing. In this case, ventilatory support must be provided until the SAB recedes. As with any RA, the potential for permanent nerve damage, while rare, is present.

## Epidural anesthesia and analgesia

The dura is the membranous tissue that encircles the spinal cord; SAB involves piercing the dura and injecting LA into the CSF. For epidural anesthesia (EA), the LA drug is injected *above* the dura, into a potential space called the epidural space. From here, the LA diffuses gradually through the dura to produce anesthesia or analgesia. Because of this gradual diffusion, the onset of anesthesia is slower than with SAB. In EA, different types, concentrations and volumes of LA are used to induce anesthesia or analgesia. Factors influencing the resulting level of analgesia or anesthesia include: the amount, type, and concentration of LA used, the area of injection, and the patient's position. Most nurses are familiar with epidural anesthesia as it is used in labor and delivery.

- Administration: With the patient sitting or lying with the back arched (to open the vertebral interspaces), the area of administration is cleansed and draped. The area chosen depends on the area where anesthesia is desired; this may be the lumbar, thoracic, or cervical area. Using a sterile technique, the anesthetist inserts a larger bore needle (usually 19 gauge) until loss of resistance is felt, indicating the epidural space has been entered. Usually a catheter is threaded through the needle for the continuous administration of LA, and the needle is subsequently removed. EA may also be a "single-shot" technique, especially when used as a treatment for chronic pain. The volume of LA administered is far greater in epidural anesthesia than in spinal anesthesia. A small "test dose" of LA is generally administered first to insure that the needle is not in a vein or the subdural space, because the injection of a large volume of LA into the circulation or the subarachnoid space could be disastrous. If the test dose is negative, the remaining LA is injected and the patient again positioned for maximum effectiveness. Because of the slower onset of EA, haste in positioning the patient is not quite as necessary as it is in SAB.

- Indications: EA is used for procedures on the abdomen and lower extremities and in treatment of chronic pain.

- Advantages: Advantages of EA include the placement of an epidural catheter which allows for additional injection of LA should the procedure take longer than necessary. There is also a wider variety of LA available for epidural anesthesia. In addition, a small dose of a narcotic can be injected through the catheter for postoperative pain relief. And unless the dura was inadvertently punctured during placement of the epidural (this is called a "wet tap"), the patient will not have a headache or need to lie flat postoperatively.

- Disadvantages: EA is not popular in ambulatory settings because of the skill required to perform the technique, the length of time to establish surgical anesthesia, and the unreliability of the LA in diffusing through the dura to produce complete anesthesia. EA can be "spotty," meaning there are some areas that are not anesthetized completely, causing distress to the patient.

- Potential complications: Hypotension isn't usually a problem with EA because the slow onset allows the body time to compensate; nevertheless, it can still occur. If the dura is inadvertently punctured during placement of the epidural ("wet tap"), a postoperative headache may develop and is usually quite severe due to the larger bore needle used in EA. If some of the LA escapes into the bloodstream, seizures or cardiac arrest could develop. If an indwelling catheter is placed, it could be inadvertently injected with drugs other than LA (with serious consequences), or part of it could break off in the tissues of the patient's back.

## Intravenous regional anesthesia

Useful for brief procedures (60-90 minutes) on the hand or foot, intravenous regional anesthesia is also called a Bier (pronounced like "beer") Block. This technique involves filling the veins of the isolated extremity with the LA xylocaine to induce anesthesia in that extremity.

- Administration: An intravenous catheter is inserted into a vein of the affected extremity, then a pneumatic tourniquet (TQ) is placed around the upper arm or ankle. The extremity is elevated and tightly wrapped with an elastic bandage to exsanguinate it, and the TQ is inflated. The elastic wrap is removed and the veins are filled with the LA xylocaine (around 40-50 cc) via the IV catheter; the TQ restricts the LA to the extremity. This induces anesthesia in the extremity while the TQ is inflated.

- Indications: IV regional anesthesia is useful in short procedures on the hand, forearm or foot of the ambulatory patient, especially simple procedures like ganglion cyst excision or carpal tunnel release.

- Advantages: IV regional anesthesia is an excellent technique for ambulatory patients because it anesthetizes only the affected area, is generally reliable, and complications are rare.

- Disadvantages: IV regional anesthesia may not be possible in some injuries, because the tight wrapping of the extremity necessary for the block can prove too painful to the patient. If the TQ is inadvertently released before the procedure ends, anesthesia will be lost. Some patients will complain of TQ pain before the procedure is complete and subsequently require general anesthesia; this may delay recovery and discharge of the ambulatory patient.

- Potential complications: Sudden release of the TQ will allow the LA to flood into the bloodstream; this large volume of LA may trigger seizures. Because of this, the TQ must be released slowly when the procedure is completed. Letting the TQ down gradually allows slow release of the LA into the bloodstream so the body can compensate.

## Nerve blocks

Skilled practitioners may inject LA into the area of specific nerves in order to induce anesthesia in that area.

- Administration: The injection site is cleaned and LA is injected around the nerve and nerve fibers that serve a particular region of the body. Examples are ankle and axillary blocks.

- Indications: Nerve blocks are used for surgery on the extremities or a specific part of the body.

- Advantages: Nerve blocks are excellent choices for ambulatory patients because the patient avoids the nausea and drowsiness that often accompany general anesthesia, and the block often affords some degree of postoperative pain relief.

- Disadvantages: Nerve blocks require technical skill and even then may not result in adequate anesthesia. The patient must be able to cooperate with the injection(s) necessary to establish the block. These blocks are often time consuming to perform, causing delays in the schedule; this is a distinct disadvantage in ambulatory care.

- Potential complications: Postoperative neuropathy is rare but possible.

# LOCAL ANESTHESIA

A simple anesthetic is the injection of LA into the area where the physician will be working. The LA infiltrates the area to produce anesthesia. Most people have experienced this type of anesthesia in their dentist's office. This is called local anesthesia, and you may hear this technique referred to as "straight local," meaning the patient will not receive any sedation or special monitoring by an anesthetist. This is most often the case in physicians' offices, minor emergency clinics, and specialty areas of a hospital. However, because the injection of local anesthetics is unpleasant, many physicians will want the patient undergoing a longer procedure to have conscious sedation; this is reviewed in the next section. Table 6-1 lists common LA used in regional and local techniques.

- Administration: The injection site is cleaned and LA is injected by the practitioner into the area where he or she will be working.

### Table 6-1
### Common Local Anesthetics

| Local Anesthetic | Common Use(s) |
| --- | --- |
| lidocaine (Xylocaine) | Local infiltration, regional anesthetics such as spinal and epidurals, nerve blocks, intravenous regional (Bier Block), topical anesthesia |
| bupivacaine (Marcaine) | Local infiltration, regional anesthetics such as spinal and epidurals, nerve blocks. Bupivacaine is a longer acting LA and can provide some postoperative pain relief. |
| chloroprocaine (Nesacaine) | Epidural analgesia and anesthesia.. |
| cocaine | Nasopharyngeal anesthesia during sinus or nasal surgery. |

- Indications: Local anesthesia is used for minor procedures such as removal of lesions or suturing wounds, although even extensive plastic surgery may be done under local anesthesia.

- Advantages: Somnolence, sedation, and postoperative nausea are not a concern when the patient receives only local anesthesia. The healthy patient having a brief minor procedure under local anesthesia also does not usually require electronic monitoring. Local anesthesia is safe and effective for many minor procedures.

- Disadvantages: Injection of LA can be painful and the patient may be uncomfortable; the patient will likely become restless during a long procedure. Nervous patients may experience intense anxiety leading to hypertension and cardiac arrhythmias.

- Potential complications: An overdosage of LA may cause a seizure; seizures or cardiovascular collapse may develop from LA toxicity. This is most often associated with injection of large amounts of LA. Bradycardia or even asystole may be triggered by the retrobulbar injection of LA around the eye for ophthalmic surgery. While true allergies to local anesthetics are rare, a reaction is possible.

# MONITORED ANESTHESIA CARE AND CONSCIOUS SEDATION

Many ambulatory procedures are performed under local anesthesia in a patient who also receives intravenous sedatives while being monitored by an anesthetist or nurse. Terminology regarding this varies, but you may hear this called "local with sedation," "local/IV," "local standby," or "conscious sedation."

Experts differ on an exact and uniform definition of conscious sedation (Burden, 1993 p. 240), but in general, conscious sedation means the administration of intravenous agents to induce drowsiness. Although sedated, the patient should continue to respond to verbal commands, maintain a patent airway, and have stable vital signs.

The American Society of Anesthesiologists has officially labelled this type of care as "monitored anesthesia care" or MAC. During MAC, an anesthetist is present to monitor the patient and provide sedation, oxygen, or other anesthesia and medical care, and to manage complications should any arise (Miller 1322). An example is a patient having a face lift. In this case, the surgeon injects the LA into the operative site, and the anesthetist administers sedatives as needed, while monitoring the patient's condition during the procedure. Whatever such care is called in your locale, it is likely that you will see more of it in ambulatory patient care in the future because, as discussed in Chapter 1, increasingly complex procedures are being shifted into the ambulatory care setting.

In some settings, the physician performing the procedure will administer intravenous sedatives or ask the nurse to do so in the absence of an anesthetist. This is an area of concern to nurses who may feel they lack the skills or the time to administer intravenous agents and adequately monitor the patient while still performing their routine nursing duties. Many institutions have addressed this difficult question by establishing policies regarding who may administer intravenous agents and who will monitor the patient receiving such drugs. In 1992, the Association of Operating Room Nurses (AORN) published a statement of recommended practices for monitoring the patient receiving IV conscious sedation; this was reprinted in the AORN Journal in 1993 p. 978 57:4. The American Nurses Association has also developed guidelines (Resource 18 Burden p. 709) for the role of the Registered Nurse in this situation. Nurses being asked to administer intravenous sedation should review these standards, assess their own professional skills and knowledge, determine the policy at their facility, and review their state's Nurse Practice Act before agreeing to administer intravenous sedation during procedures. Unfamiliarity with the drugs administered or inability to manage complications could cause patient injury or death.

### Pharmacologic agents

Some of the pharmacologic agents used for conscious sedation are briefly listed below. A more detailed discussion of each can be found in Chapter 5, General Anesthesia.

- Narcotics: Narcotics such as fentanyl (Sublimaze) may be administered to reduce the pain of local anesthetic injection. Narcotics are also administered to sedate patients, because narcotics produce an effect that many people find pleasurable.

- Tranquilizers: The benzodiazepine tranquilizers such as midazolam (Versed) or diazepam (Valium) are popular in ambulatory procedures; these drugs decrease anxiety and reduce recall of the procedure.

- Hypnotics: Drugs which induce drowsiness and unconsciousness include propofol (Diprivan), and the barbiturate sodium thiopental (Pentothal). These drugs produce this effect in a dose-dependent fashion.

- Gases: During local anesthesia with sedation, the patient usually receives oxygen; nitrous oxide ("laughing gas") may also be administered.

**Monitoring.** The patient undergoing local anesthesia with sedation should be monitored at a minimum with an electrocardiograph, precordial stethoscope, pulse oximeter, and blood pressure gauge. More extensive monitoring may be indicated based on the patient's condition and the type of procedure being performed.

# NURSING STRATEGIES FOR THE AMBULATORY PATIENT UNDERGOING REGIONAL OR LOCAL ANESTHESIA OR SEDATION

General nursing strategies for the ambulatory patient undergoing regional or local anesthesia or sedation are based on the nursing duty to: ready the patient for the procedure, prepare for untoward events, support the patient psychologically, and assess the patient's recovery. Specific nursing strategies and nursing actions can be found in Chapters 7, 8, and 9, which detail care of the ambulatory patient during the perioperative period. Table 6-2 lists several common nursing diagnoses for patients undergoing RA, LA, and conscious sedation.

General nursing strategies you can take when an ambulatory patient requires regional or local anesthesia or conscious sedation include:

- Note that the patient must still fast before RA or MAC because general anesthesia may become necessary should the block fail or the patient become too restless, or in the event a complication such as a seizure develops.

- Tell ambulatory patients that LA, RA, and MAC are routinely used in many procedures and are generally well tolerated and well accepted by patients. Patients receiving MAC usually doze

### Table 6-2
### Potential Nursing Diagnoses for Patients Undergoing Regional or Local Anesthesia or Conscious Sedation

| Nursing Diagnosis | Nursing intervention |
|---|---|
| Fear, related to unfamiliarity (with RA, LA, or MAC) | Explore patient's fears, then address those concerns or ask the anesthetist to answer them. Common fears are: fear of permanent paralysis, fear of seeing the procedure or having to watch it, fear of pain during placement of RA or injection of LA, fear of pain during the procedure. Reassure the patient that LA and RA are generally quite safe, that discomfort is minimal, that they will not have to watch the surgery; administer sedatives as ordered. If sensorimotor function is slow to return, reassure the patient that recovery times vary and most recoveries from RA are routine and uncomplicated; ask anesthetist to evaluate and reassure patient as necessary. |
| Pain, related to physical or chemical agents (LA injection or placement of RA). | Acknowledge that injection of LA may be briefly uncomfortable, but explain that a nurse will be present to comfort patient; know whether the patient will receive conscious sedation and if so, tell the patient that discomfort is usually minimal. Emphasize the positive benefits of having the procedure under RA or LA: avoidance of possible nausea and drowsiness that often follows GA. |
| Injury, potential related to sensory or motor deficits | Remind the patient having RA or LA that the anesthetized part is prone to injury until sensorimotor functions return; monitor the affected area and the environment to prevent injury; assist the patient with standing the first time after the procedure. |
| Knowledge deficit related to lack of exposure (to RA, LA, or MAC) | Give clear concise explanations, using terminology appropriate to patient's level of understanding and reinforce often; answer patient's questions about anesthesia and ask the anesthetist to reinforce your teaching and/or address the patient's concerns; establish an atmosphere of trust that will not minimize importance of the patient's concerns; provide written information as appropriate. |
| Anxiety related to situational crisis (receiving RA, LA, or MAC) | Listen to patient and allow verbalization of concerns; offer verbal reassurance and gentle touch as indicated and appropriate. Alter the environment when possible to reduce stress: reduce noise, provide privacy, minimize traffic through patient care area. |

Please note this is a sample of potential nursing diagnoses and is not presented as, nor intended to be, a complete care plan for the ambulatory patient. More complete information can be found in a medical surgical nursing course and textbook.

Adapted from: *Nursing Diagnosis Reference Manual* by Sheila Sparks and Cynthia M. Taylor, Springhouse Corporation, 1991, and *Overview of Anesthesia for Nurses* by Linda Chitwood, Western Schools, 1992.

through the procedure and remember little about it later. This helps reduce patient anxiety.

- Consider applying a small personal radio/tape player with headphones to patients during the procedure. Soft music played through the headphones helps distract the patient and reduces anxiety for many patients. (Note however that patients who wear hearing aids usually do not want to use headphones because it interferes with their hearing aid).

- Reassure the patient and support person that serious complications from RA, such as paralysis, are rare. This helps reduce patient anxiety. Many patients claim to know of someone who was paralyzed after RA; acknowledge that while such a result is possible, it in unlikely. However, the patient should know that just like any other branch of medicine, anesthesia is not an exact or perfect science.

- Emphasize the benefits of RA or LA over general anesthesia; this should increase patient acceptance. Nausea and drowsiness are minimal or nonexistent after RA or LA, and the block may afford some degree of postoperative pain relief.

- Remind the ambulatory patient that the loss of sensorimotor function after RA will render the affected area vulnerable to injury. This will increase the patient's awareness of the potential for injury and help secure the patient's cooperation in monitoring for potential injury.

- Check the labels of all local anesthetics you pass to the anesthetist or surgeon for injection of the patient. Many LA come in different strengths and formulations to match specific anesthetic techniques; this information will be stated on the label. Repeat this information from the label to the person using the drug, and offer the bottle label to them so they can verify it is the correct drug. Careful checking of LA labels can prevent failed techniques and tragic errors.

- Note that true allergies to local anesthetics are quite rare. What many patients report as an allergy is often the effect of epinephrine that may have been added to the drug. This can cause unpleasant sensations such as rapid heartbeat, dizziness, and anxiety. Tell the patient that this "allergy" may not preclude the use of a regional or local anesthetic, but insure that the anesthetist and surgeon are aware of this reported allergy so they can investigate it further.

- Know the location of emergency supplies such as airway management equipment and emergency drugs; know how to call an emergency team to the area if more help is needed. Complications from LA are rare but seconds can be critical; knowing the location of these supplies and how to get help may save the patient's life.

- Respect the patient's fears about RA or LA even if they seem trivial or are misguided; avoid belittling or laughing at expressed concerns. Acknowledging the patient's concerns as legitimate helps boost the patient's confidence in the nurse; addressing these concerns and then correcting misconceptions reduces patient anxiety.

- Exercise great caution when you are asked to administer drugs you are not familiar with or feel unqualified to give. Nurses who administer conscious sedation should have advanced training and skills because they must be prepared to manage any complications that may develop after administration.

- Note that while most regional anesthetics are completed without incident, the potential for major complications does exist, so the nurse must anticipate problems and be prepared to assist in treatment as necessary. The nurse who is able to do this can mean the difference in a good versus a bad outcome for the patient.

- Follow your institution's policy when determining street readiness for the patient who had RA, LA, or MAC. Recovery from any of these anesthesia techniques varies among patients, and discharge too early could compromise patient safety.

# SUMMARY

Regional and local anesthetic techniques hold an important place in ambulatory care; these techniques may be increasingly utilized in the future. This chapter reviewed fundamental aspects of regional and local anesthesia for the ambulatory patient. Different types of regional anesthesia were discussed; the common indications, advantages, disadvantages and potential complications of each were described. Conscious sedation, or monitored anesthesia care (MAC), was also reviewed. General nursing strategies for the patient undergoing one of these anesthetics were described.

# CRITICAL CONCEPTS

- Regional anesthesia is generally quite safe; paralysis and serious complications are rare. Nevertheless, some patients will refuse RA because of these fears.

- RA, LA, and MAC are often good alternatives to general anesthesia (GA) for the ambulatory patient because drowsiness and nausea are usually minimal or nonexistent.

- RA is not as popular as GA for the ambulatory patient because of the time and degree of skill it takes to induce and the fact that RA is not always as reliable as GA in producing anesthesia (loss of sensation).

- Nurses being asked to administer intravenous sedation should at a minimum review practice standards, assess their own professional skills and knowledge, determine the policy at their facility, and review their state's Nurse Practice Act before agreeing to administer intravenous sedation during any procedure.

- Patients scheduled to have RA or MAC must still fast in case GA becomes necessary during the procedure, or in the even that complications such as seizures develop.

# EXAM QUESTIONS

## CHAPTER 6

Questions 24-30

24. Two regional anesthetic techniques are:
    a. total and partial intravenous
    b. spinal and epidural
    c. Bier block and inhalation
    d. brain block and Bier block

25. The ambulatory patient having a SAB may have to lie flat for a period of time to help reduce the chance of postoperative:
    a. syncope
    b. paralysis
    c. headache
    d. neuropathy

26. The leak of fluid through the hole in the dura made by the spinal needle can result in a:
    a. spinal headache
    b. chemical neuropathy
    c. cerebrovascular accident
    d. distended bladder

27. One common fear patients may express about regional anesthesia is of:
    a. permanent paralysis
    b. revealing personal information
    c. losing bowel control
    d. waking up during the procedure

28. Hypotension would be most likely with which of the following RA techniques?
    a. interscatene
    b. intravenous
    c. spinal
    d. epidural

29. A severe headache may develop after epidural anesthesia if which of the following occurred during placement?
    a. wet tap
    b. hypotension
    c. affhythmias
    d. syncope

30. Inducing loss of sensation in a specific area of the body is what type of anesthesia?
    a. inhalation
    b. regional
    c. intravenous
    d. neuromuscular

# CHAPTER 7

# PREPARING THE PATIENT FOR THE PROCEDURE

## CHAPTER OBJECTIVE

After completing this chapter, you should be better prepared to plan nursing care for the patient preparing to undergo an ambulatory procedure.

## LEARNING OBJECTIVES

After reading this chapter, you should be able to:

1. Specify steps in preparing patients for ambulatory procedures.

2. Identify nursing actions that enhance the comfort and safety of the patient being prepared for an ambulatory procedure.

3. Select potential nursing diagnoses for patients being prepared for an ambulatory procedure.

4. Recognize the significance of the preanesthesia evaluation.

5. Indicate the rationale for patient fasting before certain procedures.

6. Identify medications sometimes administered before ambulatory surgery and choose nursing actions relevant to administration of those drugs.

7. Recognize the importance of preoperative teaching in ambulatory care.

8. Differentiate between perioperative team members.

## INTRODUCTION

Proper preparation of the patient for an ambulatory procedure is a key factor in the success of the procedure; nurses bear much of the burden for that preparation. This chapter discusses the role of the nurse in preparing the ambulatory patient for a planned ambulatory procedure. The pressure to work quickly, often felt in an ambulatory setting, is addressed. The perioperative team and their roles are identified. The first steps of the nursing process, assessment and planning, are reviewed. Preoperative teaching is examined, as is the preanesthesia evaluation. Preoperative medications are explored. Nursing strategies that facilitate preparation of the patient are reviewed. The chapter closes with a summary and a list of the critical concepts presented.

# PATIENT PREPARATION IN THE AMBULATORY SETTING

Health care facility administrators need maximum efficiency and return on their investment in equipment and personnel; surgeons will threaten to take their patients to another facility if they experience delays between cases (Culczynski, Fall 1993 APSF p. 28). So time is a critical factor in the cost-effectiveness of ambulatory care, and it is often a significant factor in the physician's selection of the facility for ambulatory treatment. Performing the maximum number of procedures in the least amount of time enhances cost-effectiveness; physicians are often anxious to proceed with their cases in order to avoid wasted productive time. Cost-effectiveness and physician satisfaction are enhanced when the schedule flows smoothly with a minimum of delays and with little or no inactive periods ("down time") between cases. Ambulatory surgery centers also try to minimize the time between surgical cases that it takes to prepare the operating room for the next patient ("turn around time") because this is cost-effective and appeals to surgeons. Staying on schedule is also important because delays disrupt all procedures following the delayed case. This means that subsequent patients may have to wait; patients often disapprove of this inconvenience and may experience increased anxiety while they wait. Because of these factors, ambulatory care nurses often labor under heavy pressure to prepare patients quickly for procedures. Time also limits nursing care because, by definition, the ambulatory patient will come and go during the day; the nursing process must be completed within this short time frame.

This pressure to prepare patients must neither lead to inadequate preparation nor should the patient feel like just another case moving through an impersonal system. In the first situation, such haste may lead to errors that can result in increased morbidity and mortality for the patient. In the latter, the patient suffers and does not receive the best possible care to which he or she is entitled. So the nurse preparing ambulatory patients for procedures must be well organized and efficient, always assessing the patient and constantly adapting the nursing process to the patient's needs. To become so involved in meeting the needs of the facility or physician that the patient's needs are outranked, ignored, or overlooked, is not only unfortunate but unethical. Table 7-1, from Burden (1993) p. 153 summarizes the goals of preoperative preparations.

---

**Table 7-1**
**Goals of Preoperative Preparations**

- Collection of data through assessment and interview
- Provision of accurate information to patient and family
- Assurance of appropriate preoperative compliance
- Promotion of the wellness concept
- Improving lines of communication
- Provision of emotional support
- Reduction of patient anxiety
- Decreasing potential for complications
- Provision of smooth flow of the surgery schedule

*Source*: *Ambulatory Surgical Nursing* by Nancy Burden, W. B. Saunders & Co., 1993.

---

# THE PERIOPERATIVE TEAM

Preparing the patient for an ambulatory procedure means coordinating the efforts of all the professionals involved in the planned care. Below is a brief review of those professionals and the role they have in the ambulatory patient's care.

## Nurses

Registered nurses, licensed practical or vocational nurses, and sometimes nursing assistants may comprise the patient's nursing team, although ambulatory care nurses seldom have the luxury of assistants. The Registered Nurse heads the nursing team and directs or performs preparation of the patient and also functions as the patient's advocate.

## Physicians

The patient coming for an ambulatory procedure is often being treated by a specialist, a doctor who is not their primary care physician. Examples are patients coming for radiologic studies or specialty surgery. Exceptions are women undergoing gynecologic or obstetric procedures, because these physicians often serve as a woman's primary doctor.

## Anesthesia team

Anesthesia care may be provided by either an individual or a team. That individual may be either a nurse anesthetist or a physician. A team is usually made up of a nurse anesthetist and an anesthesiologist. For the purposes of this book, the person providing anesthesia care is referred to simply as the anesthetist.

- Nurse anesthetist: Registered Nurses with advanced training who have passed a national certifying examination (board certification), who maintain certification by continuing education credits, and who meet practice requirements are called Certified Registered Nurse Anesthetists (CRNA). Nurses first specialized in the administration of anesthesia over a century ago (Fraulini, 1987).

- Anesthesiologists: Physicians with advanced formal training in the administration of anesthesia are called anesthesiologists, but not all physicians who administer anesthesia have completed such training. While nurses are required to maintain national certification to administer anesthesia, physicians are not.

## Ancillary personnel

In some cases, the patient has laboratory and other diagnostic exams performed outside the facility; those results may be forwarded to the ambulatory facility. In other facilities, ambulatory care nurses draw blood and obtain urine specimens, then actually run the tests themselves in the facility and place the results on the patient's chart. In other units, usually ambulatory units connected with hospitals, technicians draw blood or run electrocardiograms. Ambulatory surgery facilities often employ trained technicians to scrub and assist the surgeon in surgery; some doctors employ their own assistants to help in surgery and patient care.

# PATIENT PREPARATION: ASSESSMENT AND PLANNING

As described in Chapter 3, the nursing process helps in organizing and delivering nursing care, especially in the time sensitive environment of ambulatory care. The first two steps of the nursing process, assessment and planning, are utilized in the preparation of the patient for ambulatory care. Accurate assessment can be a pivotal factor in the ambulatory patient's safety; planning is essential to efficient care and influences the outcome of that care.

Under ideal circumstances, the physician who prescribes an ambulatory procedure assesses the patient's fitness and identifies concerns that must be considered in that patient's care: chronic disease, regular medications that may influence the choice of preprocedure diagnostic testing or anesthesia, and the patient's suitability for ambulatory care. However, the ideal seldom exists in the real world. Often the physician is not the patient's primary doctor, and this doctor may be unaware of the patient's complete medical history. Another ideal standard recommends that the patient visit the facility a day or two before a major or invasive ambulatory procedure such as surgery. This reduces time pressure on the day of the procedure and affords you an opportunity to alert other team members of any concerns or potential problems. It also gives the patient a chance to observe the facility and ask questions; this generally reduces patient anxiety. However, patients may resist making two trips to the facility, and it may prove a hardship for the patient coming from out of town. As a result, many patients will not be seen by the ambulatory care nurse until the day of the procedure. A few facilities require an ambulatory patient to come for a preadmission interview; some compromise by having the nurse contact the patient by telephone to begin the assessment, identify concerns, and give preprocedure instructions such as fasting.

However the nursing assessment is begun, it forms the foundation for the care delivered by the ambulatory team not just the nurse. Physicians, anesthetists, and others often seek the record of the nurse's admission assessment first, because of the wealth of information found there. If this foundation is weak or inaccurate, patient care may suffer. During nursing assessment of the patient, be careful to provide privacy during the interview and physical exam. Note that some patients may prefer for their support person to wait in another room during this time. Nursing assessment of the ambulatory patient includes:

## Reason for admission

Ascertain that the patient understands why he or she is at the facility. The patient should be able to state why he or she is there and what treatment is expected. In a few cases, as with young children or perhaps an Alzheimer's patient, you may have to turn to the guardian for this information.

## Review of body systems and current health status

A precise review of the patient's prior health history highlights potential problem areas and helps the team plan care to minimize the chance of complications. Review the major body systems such as the cardiovascular or musculoskeletal systems and ask the patient about major illnesses, serious accidents, and hospitalizations. All female patients of childbearing age should be asked about the possibility of pregnancy; some facilities require a negative pregnancy test before a procedure. Document any reactions the patient or family may have had to anesthesia. While many patients will report nausea or vomiting after anesthesia, there is an anesthetic complication known as Malignant Hyperthermia that runs in families (see Chapter 14). This rare but serious complication must be reported immediately to the anesthetist; the scheduled procedure may have to be cancelled in order to allow a thorough evaluation and intensive planning for an anesthetic.

## List of all medications

Include nicotine and recreational alcohol or illicit drug use. Many patients don't consider over-the-counter or illicit drugs reportable, but these drugs can interact with anesthetics or adversely affect operating conditions. For example, aspirin or non-steroidal anti-inflammatory agents such as ibuprofen (Motrin) can inhibit clotting; cocaine can cause fatal arrhythmias when epinephrine is injected or certain anesthetic agents are used. Document alcohol and tobacco use by asking the patient to estimate the amount consumed: "How many cigarettes do you smoke in an average day?"

## Allergies

Note allergies the patient claims to food and drugs; also note key symptoms the patient claims result from exposure to these allergens, such as wheezing or itching. This can help distinguish true allergies from common unpleasant side effects.

## Social history

You should note the patient's level of education and understanding of the procedure, employment, and support system for aftercare. This information will help in identifying potential needs during and after the procedure.

## Emotional status

Report the patient's anxiety level; do not assume that because the patient is ambulatory that emotional distress will be minimal (Sheperd, 1990 JPAN, Vol. 5 No. 2 April p. 103-105). Assess the level of support offered by the person accompanying the patient. If the patient is required to have someone drive him or her home, verify that the patient has made such plans. Assessment of the patient's support system is important in ambulatory care because the support person in many cases must assume responsibility for aftercare that otherwise would have been provided by a nurse.

## Prosthetics

Record the presence of dentures, caps, bridges, partial plates, and other dental devices. Artificial dental appliances are seldom as strong as the original structures, so the team needs to identify these areas; this information is useful in the event airway management equipment must be inserted into the mouth, and as a medicolegal issue in case the patient claims the teeth were damaged during the procedure. Note whether the patient has contact lens these should be removed before general anesthesia. Inquire about other artificial parts such as wigs or limbs. This will help you plan care and helps your team avoid surprises during the delivery of care.

## Time of last oral intake

Note the time of last oral intake; remember that some patients don't consider gum, mints, or water as oral intake. Remind the patient of the importance of NPO, and then be certain that you have the correct time of last intake by repeating it to the patient for verification. Notify the physician and anesthetist immediately if the patient has been non-compliant, because the procedure may need to be rescheduled or cancelled.

## Height and weight

Obtain these measurements yourself when possible; avoid accepting the patient's stated weight, because some patients may not know or will not divulge their correct weight. These parameters help the anesthetist plan care, because drug dosages and equipment used (such as endotracheal tubes) are based on body size. Certain conditions such as obesity also can necessitate adaptations in the anesthetist's care plan. Record the patient's height also; this reveals information about the amount and degree of obesity or malnutrition.

## Physical exam

Perform a brief physical exam, noting the patient's skin color, venous access, edema of extremities if present, and muscle weakness if any. Auscultate the heart and lungs to determine if the heart sounds are regular and the lungs clear; notify the other team members of any aberrations. Note any injuries or deficits the patient exhibits. Identify signs of anxiety such as trembling, crying, fidgeting, pacing, hesitant or rapid speech, talkativeness, hypervigilance and scanning, or sweating; record symptoms of anxiety as stated by the patient. This information helps you plan care and also serves to document the patient's

**MID SOUTH SURGERY CENTER**
**PREOP/ADMISSION RECORD**

| BP | PULSE | RESP | TEMP | WT(LB) | WT( KG) | HT | LMP | SHOE SZ | EMOTIONAL LEVEL __ CALM __ ANXIOUS __ DEPRESSED |
|---|---|---|---|---|---|---|---|---|---|

| VALUABLES YES NO | GIVEN TO | LOCKED UP | FORM SIGNED YES NO | VERBALIZED UNDERSTANDING OF PREOP TEACHING ___ |
|---|---|---|---|---|
| PERSON TO DRIVE PT HOME: | | CAREGIVER | ASSISTANCE/NEEDS AFTER DISCHARGE | |

PRE OP MEDS:

| DAILY MEDICATIONS | MEDICAL HISTORY | PREVIOUS SURGERY | ALLERGIES |
|---|---|---|---|
| | | | |
| | | | |
| | | | |
| | | | |
| | | | ALLERGY ID: |

| PREVIOUS ANESTHETIC HISTORY | FAMILY ANESTHETIC HISTORY |
|---|---|

| SMOKE | DENT APP | CONTACTS | HEAR AID | PROS DEV | ID BRACELET | SIGNED CONSENT | NPO SINCE |
|---|---|---|---|---|---|---|---|

| SURGICAL PREP SOLUTION | SITE | COMPLETED BY |
|---|---|---|

| IV START: a.m. p.m. | SITE: | GAUGE: | SOLUTION: | LOCAL: | AMT: | BY: |
|---|---|---|---|---|---|---|

| REVIEW OF SYSTEMS | | | |
|---|---|---|---|
| CARDIOVASCULAR | NEG | POS FOR | NURSES NOTES: |
| RESPIRATORY | NEG | POS FOR | |
| NEUROLOGIC | NEG | POS FOR | |
| OTHER | NEG | POS FOR | |
| PHYSICAL EXAM | | | |
| HEENT | WNL | POS FOR | |
| TEETH/MANDIBLE | WNL | POS FOR | |
| HEART | WNL | POS FOR | |
| LUNGS | WNL | POS FOR | |
| ABDOMEN | WNL | POS FOR | |
| EXTREMITIES | WNL | POS FOR | |

| PT CLEARED FOR SURGERY | GEN | MAC | EPIDURAL | LOCAL | REG | OTHER |
|---|---|---|---|---|---|---|

ASA LEVEL: 1 2 3 4 5

| ADMITTING DIAGNOSIS: | PROPOSED SURGERY |
|---|---|
| DISCHARGE DIAGNOSIS: | |

COMMENTS

| SURGEON: | ANESTHESIA: | RN: | OP REPORT DICTATED |
|---|---|---|---|

**Figure 7-1.** Sample Ambulatory Record. *Source:* Mid South Surgery Center

### Table 7-2
### Potential Nursing Diagnoses for Patients Preparing for an Ambulatory Procedure

| Nursing Diagnosis | Nursing intervention |
|---|---|
| Infection, potential related to invasive procedure | Check white blood cell count and temperature and notify perioperative team if elevated. Teach patient and support person about dressing changes postoperatively if indicated; instruct in the importance of hand washing. |
| Aspiration, potential related to surgery and anesthesia | Instruct in rationale for NPO and verify that instructions were followed; notify the other team members if not. Administer aspiration prophylaxis as ordered. |
| Powerlessness related to health care environment | Explain what you are doing and why, what to expect during and after the procedure, allow patient to make decisions whenever possible. Make time for the patient and family to ask questions and receive answers. |
| Knowledge deficit related to lack of exposure (to ambulatory care) | Orient patient to the surroundings and the expected events during care. Encourage patient and support person to ask questions when they do not understand anything that is happening. Give clear concise explanations, using terminology appropriate to level of understanding; provide written information as appropriate. Follow your teaching with an assessment of the degree of learning by the patient and review any areas where learning is incomplete. |
| Anxiety related to situational crisis (undergoing an ambulatory procedure) | Listen to the patient's concerns and help him or her identify the major factors that are at the root of the anxiety. Offer verbal reassurance and gentle touch as indicated to help calm. Speak softly and alter the environment when possible to reduce stress: reduce noise and provide privacy. Administer sedatives as ordered. Assess for concerns regarding self-concepts that may be altered by surgery such as with a breast biopsy or orthopedic surgery and address these issues. |
| Fear, related to unfamiliarity (with ambulatory care) | Establish an atmosphere where the patient feels safe. Explore patient and support person's fears, then address those concerns. Accept the patient's expressed fears as real for him or her; never belittle or ridicule patient concerns because this can increase fear and anxiety and destroy trust or confidence in the nurse. |
| Grieving, anticipatory related to potential loss (ex: D & C for incomplete abortion) | Allow patient to express concerns, do not minimize or negate feelings. Ask what you or support person can do to help (ex: hold hand, hug, sit quietly with patient). Encourage expression of feelings. Refer the patient to appropriate resources for aftercare if indicated. |

Please note this is a sample of potential nursing diagnoses and is not presented as, nor intended to be, a complete care plan for the ambulatory patient. More complete information can be found in a medical surgical nursing course and textbook.

Adapted from: *Nursing Diagnosis Reference Manual* by Sheila Sparks and Cynthia M. Taylor, Springhouse Corporation, 1991, and *Overview of Anesthesia* for Nurses by Linda Chitwood, Western Schools, 1992.

condition before the procedure in the event that any medicolegal issues later arise.

> **Table 7-3**
> **Steps to Planning Nursing Care**
>
> - Assign priorities to the nursing diagnoses
> - Establish expected outcomes (goals)
> - Select appropriate nursing actions (interventions)
> - Document the nursing diagnoses, expected outcomes, nursing interventions, and evaluations on the care plan.
>
> *From: Nursing Diagnosis Reference Manual* by Sheila Sparks and Cynthia M. Taylor, Springhouse Corporation, 1991. p. 15

### Baseline vital signs

Assessment would be incomplete without these parameters; knowing what is "normal" for the patient helps the team provide care during the perioperative period.

Now evaluate the results of any laboratory or diagnostic studies, place them on the correct patient's chart, and notify the physician or other team members of any variances that might require their attention. With the assessment complete, you should document your findings. See Figure 7-1 for a sample ambulatory record that incorporates the nursing and anesthesia assessments. (Mid South Surgery Center)

Using the information from the assessment and diagnostic studies, you are now ready to formulate nursing diagnoses and begin to plan care based on those identified patient needs. Some common nursing diagnoses for the preoperative patient are reviewed in Table 7-2. This is by no means a complete list; you may identify more, less, or different needs for your patient.

### Planning

The assessment leads to the formulation of the nursing diagnoses; the diagnoses guide you in planning care for your patient. Once you are familiar with common nursing diagnoses for ambulatory patients, you will find planning care is easier and more efficient because you are aware of common concerns and potential pitfalls. All that remains is to tailor your plan to meet the patient's needs. Table 7-3 reviews the four steps to planning care.

# PREOPERATIVE & PREPROCEDURE TEACHING

Informational needs were found to be the highest priority for families in the perioperative period (Carmody, Hickey, & Bookbinder, 1991 AORN J 54:3 p. 561 Sept.). These nurse researchers found that families were better able to provide support for patients if they were well informed. Nursing researchers Leino-Kilpi & Buorenheimo (1993 AORN J. May 57:5 p. 1061) also showed that patients had a strong need for information. Ideally, dissemination of information about the disorder and proposed procedure should begin in the physician's office when the procedure is scheduled. The physician should explain why the procedure is necessary, how it will be performed, the potential risks and benefits, NPO (if necessary), and any required diagnostic preprocedure testing. Realistically though, nurses bear the majority of the burden for teaching patients about the procedure and what to expect during the perioperative period. And patient teaching is not a luxury but may be required by the accrediting institution, such as the Joint Commission on Accreditation of Hospitals (McCormick & Gilson-Parkevich, 1979 p. 8).

## Teaching and learning

Teaching means to present information to another for learning; learning means to acquire knowledge or skill. The methods of teaching most commonly used in ambulatory care include: one-on-one lecture; demonstration, practice, and return demonstrations; and visual aids such as videotapes that are either viewed in the facility or sent to the patient's home (Yale, 1993 AORN J May 57:4 p. 901-908), or handouts. For learning to occur, the environment must be prepared for the learner (patient), and the patient must be ready to learn. A patient overwhelmed with pain or anxiety is not ready to learnthese concerns must be addressed first. The material to be taught must be presented at the learner's level of understanding. Knowing the patient's prior medical history, educational level, and type of employment facilitate teaching because you have greater insight of the patient's prior experiences and ability to grasp abstract or complex concepts. Evaluate the patient's degree of learning by posing questions or requesting return demonstrations.

## Content

Note that a number of books are available on patient teaching so that you do not always have to engineer a complete teaching plan for each patient. These resources can enhance your understanding of the teaching and learning process and facilitate patient teaching; some references include sample teaching and information sheets that may be distributed to patients. While it would be impossible to list all learning needs for all ambulatory patients, here are some common learning needs of ambulatory patients being prepared for a procedure:

- What to expect before the procedure, including preparation for the procedure and diagnostic studies that may be performed.

- Who will be involved in providing care before and during the procedure; who will be leading the team (Ex: surgeon, radiologist). The support person should also know who will be responsible for relaying information to him or her while the patient is undergoing the procedure.

- What sensations may be experienced, including sights, sounds, and painful stimuli; how long the procedure usually takes.

Note that it is not the nurse's obligation or role to speculate for the patient on the possible results of surgery. Questions specific to surgery should generally be deferred to the surgeon. For example, if an orthopedic surgery patient asks you whether or not the operation will restore full use of her knee, you should explain that the surgeon is the one qualified to answer that question.

## Documentation

While a significant amount of patient teaching goes on everyday in health care facilities, it is often not documented, possibly because it is time-consuming to write such narrative notes in the patient's chart. Many facilities have resolved this by putting check-off boxes on the nurse's notes to indicate that teaching was performed. Cordell and Smith-Blair (1994 Nursing 94 Vol. 24 No. 1 p. 57-59) propose a documentation form that doesn't require extensive notation yet covers the information being taught and the patient's response. Innovations like these should help the nurse plan, organize, and document teaching for the ambulatory patient.

# PREANESTHESIA EVALUATION

All patients undergoing general or regional anesthesia, or intravenous sedation with monitored anesthesia care (MAC) should be evaluated before the procedure by a member of the anesthesia team. The preanesthesia evaluation includes a patient interview to gather information, a brief physical examination, and presentation of the anesthesia plan to the patient for his or her consent.

## Preanesthesia interview

The purpose of the preanesthesia interview is to gather information about the patient's medical and surgical history, the current complaint, previous experiences with anesthesia, family history with anesthesia, health habits, medications, and prosthetics. Because this information forms the basis for anesthesia care during the procedure, it should be completed accurately regardless of time constraints.

- Medical and surgical history: Medical problems or surgeries may influence the type of anesthesia or agents administered to the patient. For example, a patient who has had a cervical fusion may be difficult to intubate. A patient with rheumatoid arthritis may require special attention to positioning or padding body parts during the procedure. Any system dysfunction like diabetes, heart disease, or asthma must be noted because it could affect anesthesia care.

- Current complaint: The reason why the patient is having the procedure may influence the type of anesthesia and is basic knowledge essential to the anesthetist planning care.

- Previous anesthetic experiences: Any untoward reactions or unpleasant experiences with anesthesia need to be explored in order to plan anesthetic care and address the patient's concerns. Some patients have not had an anesthetic since the days of ether and are concerned about receiving it (ether is no longer in use). Others report prolonged nausea and vomiting (N & V) after anesthesia. These patients can be reassured that new agents make nausea and vomiting less likely, but should know that some procedures are simply associated with higher incidences of N & V. Women seem to be more prone to N & V than men. Other patients, usually women, will relate a fear of having the anesthesia mask on their face; they feel like they are suffocating. These patients can be reassured that such is not the case and measures to reduce this fear can be taken.

- Family experience with anesthesia: The anesthetist asks about blood relative's reactions to anesthesia in order to identify patients who are at risk for developing malignant hyperthermia, a rare but often fatal reaction to anesthesia (see Chapter 14). Another inherited trait is an abnormal pseudocholinesterase level; this influences the type of neuromuscular blocking agent used.

- Health habits: The patient's health habits reveal much about his or her physical status. For example, a patient who cannot walk up a flight of stairs without shortness of breath may have a severely compromised circulatory system. The smoker of 2 packs of cigarettes a day will have chronically irritated airways and most likely a productive cough. This chronic irritation increases the possibility of a laryngospasm causing airway obstruction during the anesthetic period. Smoking cessation before a procedure will free up red blood cells to carry oxygen to the tissues, cells that previously carried carbon monoxide. Because nicotine constricts vessels, nicotine cessation can speed tissue healing after surgery. A referral to a smoking cessation group is appropriate for the patient who indicates a willingness to stop smoking.

- Medications: A candid discussion of any drugs (prescription, over-the-counter, or illicit) the patient uses is essential to a safe anesthetic, because as mentioned earlier, some drugs can interact with anesthetics. Note that a few patients who consistently claim to be unable to void for a urinalysis may be attempting to avoid detection of illicit substance use.

- Prosthetics: As mentioned earlier, the anesthetist should be aware of all artificial devices on the patient's body. Ambulatory patients are sometimes allowed to leave their dentures in place if endotracheal intubation is not planned because the dentures help the anesthesia mask fit better on the face. Artificial devices such as hair pins and contact lenses should be removed because after the patient is unconscious or heavily sedated he or she won't be able to say that the lens is scratching their eye or the hairpin is lacerating their scalp. All dental problems and artificial dental appliances must be noted; this aids in airway management and documents their status in the event the patient later claims the teeth or appliances were damaged during anesthesia.

## Physical examination

A brief physical examination is conducted to confirm the patient's condition and identify any potential problem areas. Below are some of the major areas of focus during the exam.

- Head and neck: The head, neck and temporomandibular joint should have full range-of-motion in order to facilitate airway management.

- Heart and lungs: The breath sounds should be clear, but any adventitious sounds may require further investigation.

- Extremities: The arms and legs are surveyed because limited range of motion could make positioning difficult in the operating room or if a regional anesthetic is planned. Preoperative complaints of pain in joints or extremities are noted so the affected area can be protected during the procedure and also to document the preoperative complaint for the record. Any potential difficulty in establishing venous access is noted as this time.

## Anesthesia care plan

After examining and interviewing the patient, the anesthetist formulates a tentative plan for anesthesia. The final choice of technique will be determined by several factors, including the patient's and surgeon's preference, the type of procedure being performed, and the patient's condition. The anesthetist may propose this plan to the patient, along with a discussion of the risks and benefits of the proposed anesthetic. This discussion can be done in a compassionate and kind manner that does not alarm the patient unnecessarily. Patient consent (or refusal) is then secured. In most cases, a patient under the age of 18 must have a parent or legal guardian give consent. The patient should then be given an opportunity to ask questions about the proposed anesthetic care plan.

# PREANESTHESIA MEDICATION

The practice of administering sedatives or other agents before anesthesia or a special procedure varies widely from one ambulatory unit to another. Common reasons for administering medication to the patient before anesthesia, surgery, or a special procedure are to allay anxiety, to reduce the potential for N & V, to reduce the risk of aspiration, and to protect the patient against abnormal responses such as bradycardia during the procedure or anesthetic. In some facilities, the anesthetist evaluates the patient in the preoperative holding area and administers sedatives or other drugs as indicated; the holding area nurse monitors the patient after this sedation and until the patient is transferred to the procedure suite. Table 7-4 lists common preanesthesia medica-

### Table 7-4
### Common Preanesthesia Medications

| Drug Classification | Use in Preanesthesia Medication | Examples |
|---|---|---|
| Tranquilizers & Antinauseants | Allay anxiety, sedation, reduce nausea | **Benzodiazepines:** midazolam (Versed), diazepam (Valium), lorazepam (Ativan)<br>**Phenothiazines:** hydroxyzine (Vistaril), promethazine (Phenergan), also has antinausea effect<br>**Butyrophenones:** droperidol (Inapsine), also has antinausea effect |
| Narcotics | Analgesia, sedation | Morphine, meperidine (Demerol), fentanyl (Sublimaze), alfentanil (Alfenta) |
| Agonist-antagonists | Analgesia, sedation | Nalbuphine (Nubain), butorphanol (Stadol), Usually less respiratory depression than with opioid narcotics |
| Barbiturates | Sedation | Pentobarbital (Nembutal), secobarbital (Seconal) |
| Anticholinergics | Reduce tracheobronchial and oral secretions, reduce bradycardia | **Belladonna compounds:** atropine, scopolamine (Transderm Scop, for postop nausea and vomiting)<br>**Synthetic:** glycopyrrolate (Robinul) |
| Histamine H$_2$ receptor antagonists | Aspiration prophylaxis | Cimetidine (Tagamet), ranitidine (Zantac) |
| Antacids | Aspiration prophylaxis | **Clear, non-particulate:** sodium citrate (Bicitra)<br>**Other:** magnesia and alumina oral suspension (Maalox) |
| GI stimulants | Aspiration prophylaxis | Metoclopramide (Reglan) |

tions; a brief overview of each classification follows. Chapter 5, General Anesthesia, describes these drugs in greater detail.

## Tranquilizers

Tranquilizers are administered before surgery and special procedures to reduce anxiety and in some cases, to reduce the potential for N & V after the procedure. The ambulatory care nurse may be asked to give these drugs intramuscularly (IM), or the dose may be injected intravenously (IV) by the anesthetist in the patient preparation area. Some tranquilizers cause prolonged drowsiness and so may be avoided in some ambulatory units.

## Aspiration prophylaxis

The risk of aspiration, where the stomach contents are inhaled into the lungs, is ever present; this serious or fatal complication is best prevented. Some facilities routinely administer antacids and histamine blockers that increase the stomach pH. The increased pH can help reduce damage to the lungs if aspiration does occur. Other ambulatory units include a GI stimulant such as metoclopramide (Reglan) that hastens emptying of the stomach's contents, so there is less to aspirate. Aspiration prophylaxies is an area under active research; watch for changes in protocols. Chapter 14 addresses the complication of aspiration.

## Narcotics

Opioid analgesics are administered before a procedure to reduce pain during the procedure and to sedate the patient. Some patients experience a euphoria from narcotics and this helps them feel relaxed and less anxious.

## Antiemetics

Nausea and vomiting are unfortunately relatively common in ambulatory patients. Prophylactic administration of antinauseants is routine in some facilities.

## Anticholinergics

In the past, anticholinergic administration before anesthesia was routine. These drugs reduce tracheobronchial and salivary secretions and prevent the bradycardia that may develop during some procedures. New anesthetic agents and techniques lessen the need for anticholinergics, although these agents are still in use in many facilities. The anticholinergic scopolamine (Transderm Scop) helps reduce N & V, especially when associated with motion sickness; it may be helpful in ambulatory care.

## Antibiotics

Many orthopedic and podiatric surgeons prescribe antibiotics before surgery; antibiotics are also indicated in the prophylaxis against bacterial endocarditis in certain patients at risk for this disorder. Administration should be started with sufficient time to complete the infusion before the tourniquet is inflated in podiatric or orthopedic surgery. This insures adequate circulation of the drug to all tissues before incision.

# NURSING STRATEGIES

The strategies for preparing an ambulatory patient for a procedure are complex and numerous; detailed information can be found in medical surgical and ambulatory care textbooks. Below, however, are basic nursing strategies and the rationale behind each. These should prove helpful as you prepare a patient for an ambulatory procedure. As always, your intervention should be within the scope of your institution's practice guidelines, and/or your state's Nurse Practice Act, as well as commensurate with your skills and training.

- Determine that the female patient of childbearing age, even a teenager, is not pregnant before administering any medication to her. Medications such as the benzodiazepine diazepam (Valium) can have teratogenic (cause malformation) effects on the fetus.

- Reassure patients who become frightened, anxious, or hesitant about the procedure. Do not insist that a reluctant patient go through with a procedure; notify the patient's doctor to resolve the situation. Do note however, that many patients are simply experiencing the anxiety commonly associated with undergoing a special procedure; compassion and reassurance will often diminish that anxiety and facilitate completion of the procedure.

- Administer medications as close to the ordered time as possible so peak effectiveness will be achieved.

- Use this quick method to convert pounds to kilograms without a calculator: Divide the patient's weight in half, then subtract the first number if the result is two digits, the first two numbers if the halved weight is three digits. Example: the patient weighs 180 lb. 180 divided by 2 is 90, then subtract 9, and the result is 81 kilograms (kg). Example: the patient weighs 250 lbs. Divide by 2 = 125, then subtract 12 to get 113 kg. (source unknown).

- Provide privacy when weighing a patient and avoid announcing this figure to others; many patients are sensitive about their weight, and making this number public can cause embarrassment and pain to the patient, even in the presence of close family members.

- Common variances in laboratory studies that may require further investigation before the patient undergoes ambulatory surgery include: white blood cell count too high (infection?) or too low (blood disorder or chronic illness?), hematocrit too low (anemia?) or much too high (blood disorder or chronic illness?), platelets too low (clotting disorder?). Chemistry studies with aberrations in sodium or potassium indicate an electrolyte imbalance that can be associated with certain medications or illness; factors in a urinalysis that require attention include blood, protein, glucose or bacteria present in the urine. Knowing which abnormal test results may delay or cancel surgery helps you practice more efficiently. For example, surgery on a patient with a potassium of 2.8 would most likely be cancelled until the potassium can be raised, but the patient with a cholesterol level of 250 would most likely receive counselling and further evaluation after surgery.

- Avoid specifying absolute time frames to the family of the surgical patient, because delays can occur or the surgery may simply take longer than planned. If the nurse specifies that the surgery will only take one hour and then it takes two, the family may experience heightened anxiety. You can say that the surgery is booked for one hour, but point out that sometimes surgery takes longer or is completed sooner depending on the surgeon's findings and the patient's condition.

- Prepare the environment to maximize patient learning, because it is difficult for a patient to learn while a technician draws blood from one arm and the admitting clerk pushes papers to be signed at the other arm. A quiet unhurried atmosphere allows the patient to focus on your instructions and request clarification as needed.

- Give the patient written information that reinforces your teaching, because the patient and support person are unlikely to be able to remember everything that you tell them, and the written information acts as a reference, a resource, and a documentation of instructions given.

- Monitor the patient carefully after administering sedation in order to detect potential complications from the medication. Raise the siderails to prevent a patient fall and place a call button within reach. In a single room preoperative holding area, leave the drapes open around the patient to facilitate observation. Begin pulse oximetry monitoring if available, because this mon-

- itor gives an audible confirmation that the patient's oxygen saturation appears to be adequate.

- Check frequently on the patient who has received sedation or other preoperative medication. Early recognition of a reaction or untoward response could avert tragedy.

- Instruct the patient in NPO, and stress that gum, mints, and water are included in the prohibition against oral intake. Because many patients believe that the rationale for NPO is to reduce postoperative nausea and vomiting, explain that the fast is necessary because anything in the stomach could come back up under anesthesia and be inhaled into the lungs, causing a serious or fatal pneumonia. Explain that chewing gum or mints stimulates the production of gastric acid and so must be avoided.

- Note that some researchers are now suggesting that NPO requirements may not be necessary in all cases; check your facility's policy and work within it or propose changes based on current standards and research. This helps insure patient safety and safe practice.

- Incorporate healthy lifestyle habits in your preoperative teaching whenever possible. Teaching patients about the value of smoking cessation, regular exercise, healthy diets, limiting or eliminating recreational drug use such as alcohol or illicit drugs can improve the patient's health. Be aware of community resources such as smoking cessation or weight management groups so you can refer patients as necessary. As health care providers, nurses would be remiss if they did not attempt to facilitate a patient's transition to a healthier lifestyle.

- Do not administer sedatives to the patient until the consent is signed and all permits are in order, because if consents are signed after the patient is sedated the legality can be questioned.

- Check with the physician and anesthetist about continuation of routine home medications during the fast or in the perioperative period. Many professionals believe that essential medications such as anti-hypertensives or cardiotonic agents should continue uninterrupted in the perioperative period. This helps to maintain steady pharmacologic activity and helps keep the patient stable during this perioperative time. These medications can be swallowed with a sip (30 cc) of water at the regularly scheduled times. The risks associated with such small oral intake are believed to be outweighed by the benefits of continuing the medication uninterrupted.

- Note that NPO is usually required even if the patient is scheduled for regional anesthesia or sedation. This is because the block might be unsuccessful, the patient might become too restless, or rare complications such as a seizure could require respiratory support. In this case, the patient is at risk for aspiration, and NPO reduces that possibility.

- Remember that a patient who has "quit" smoking but is using a prescription nicotine (Habitrol and others) transdermal patch is still receiving nicotine. Nicotine's effects include vasoconstriction with increased heart rate and blood pressure; removal of the patch can precipitate nicotine withdrawal. Applaud this patient's efforts at smoking cessation and encourage him or her to follow the prescribing physician's orders regarding tapering off and discontinuing the nicotine patches in order to experience the full benefit of smoking cessation.

- Help insure that the right patient goes for the right procedure with the right physician and the right chart and right lab reports by double-checking the chart, consent, lab reports, and wrist band. Ask the patient to verbally verify his or her name, doctor, and anticipated procedure. Double-checking helps avoid serious errors.

- Avoid letting time constraints push you into careless haste when preparing a patient for an ambulatory procedure, because this is a potential threat to a safe outcome and often increases the patient's anxiety.

- Follow your facility's policy or the anesthetist's orders about removal of dentures and contact lenses before a procedure. Contact lenses left in place during general anesthesia can scratch the cornea and damage the eye. Dentures and other dental appliances may become loose and be lost, or worse, obstruct the airway.

## SUMMARY

This chapter discussed the role of the nurse in preparing the ambulatory patient for a planned ambulatory procedure. The pressure to work quickly, often felt in an ambulatory setting, was addressed. The perioperative team and their roles were identified. The first steps of the nursing process, assessment and planning, were reviewed. Preoperative teaching was examined, as was the preanesthesia evaluation. Preoperative medications were briefly explored. Nursing strategies to prepare the ambulatory patient for a procedure were reviewed.

## CRITICAL CONCEPTS

- Ambulatory care nurses must be efficient time managers with sharp assessment skills and the ability to teach both the patient and support person.

- Intense pressure to get ambulatory patients through the system as quickly as possible can lead to haste and serious error.

- Essential medications such as anti-hypertensive or cardiotonic drugs are often continued during the perioperative period so that homeostasis will be maintained; these medications can be given with a sip of water if the anesthetist's policy permits.

- Patients must usually be NPO for any type of anesthesia care because of the potential need for airway management in the event of complications.

- The need for emotional support and care is not reduced in the ambulatory patient.

# EXAM QUESTIONS

## Chapter 7

Questions 31-44

31. Patients must fast before surgery and other special procedures to reduce the risk of:

    a. hyperthermia
    b. nausea
    c. rigors
    d. aspiration ✓

32. The four basic steps to planning nursing care for the ambulatory patient include assigning priorities, establishing expected outcomes, selecting nursing actions, and:

    a. documenting the process ✓
    b. ordering necessary supplies
    c. auscultating the lungs
    d. performing a physical exam

33. The preanesthesia interview forms the basis for what during the procedure?

    a. anesthesia care ✓
    b. surgeon's procedure
    c. ORT's setup procedure
    d. discharge planning

34. A common nursing diagnosis for the ambulatory surgery patient is:

    a. altered protection
    b. diversional activity deficit
    c. dysreflexia
    d. fear ✓

35. A high priority for preoperative surgical patients and their families is:

    a. information ✓
    b. rest
    c. nutrition
    d. fear

36. An assistant scrubbing on a surgical case may be employed by the facility or the:

    a. patient
    b. nurse
    c. physician ✓
    d. administrator

37. A nurse who has qualified to administer anesthesia is a:

    a. CRNA ✓
    b. LVN
    c. CNM
    d. NP

38. Ranitidine (Zantac) or cimetidine (Tagamet) may be administered before surgery to reduce the incidence of:

    a. aspiration ✓
    b. bradycardia
    c. hypertension
    d. syncope

# CHAPTER 7 - AMBULATORY PATIENT CARE

39. Gum and mints are also forbidden during patient fasting (NPO) because they can:

    a. cause nausea postoperatively
    b. prolong bleeding times
    c. stimulate gastric acid production
    d. slow bowel transit times

40. Midazolam may be administered before the procedure to reduce:

    a. nausea
    b. pain
    c. blood pressure
    d. anxiety

41. Meperidine (Demerol) may be administered before the procedure to sedate the patient and relieve:

    a. pain
    b. nausea
    c. hypotension
    d. colitis

42. Transdermal scopolamine (Transderm-Scop) is applied before surgery to reduce the postoperative incidence of:

    a. nausea and vomiting
    b. orthostatic hypotension
    c. pain and headache
    d. syncope and trauma

43. A drug that hastens emptying of the stomach is:

    a. metoclopramide (Reglan)
    b. meperidine (Demerol)
    c. propofol (Diprivan)
    d. secobarbital (Seconal)

44. The infusion should be completed before the tourniquet is inflated for which of the following types of drugs:

    a. barbiturates
    b. opioids
    c. antibiotics
    d. anticholinergics

# CHAPTER 8

# NURSING CARE OF THE PATIENT DURING THE PROCEDURE

## CHAPTER OBJECTIVE

After completing this chapter, you should be better prepared to implement nursing care for your patient during an ambulatory care procedure.

## LEARNING OBJECTIVES

After reading this chapter, you should be able to:

1. Recognize potential nursing diagnoses of ambulatory patients during the procedure.

2. Identify nursing actions that contribute to a safe and effective outcome of an ambulatory procedure.

3. Specify nursing actions that enhance the comfort of the patient during the procedure.

4. Identify monitors routinely used during ambulatory procedures.

5. Select methods to help keep patients warm during surgery.

## INTRODUCTION

The goal of nursing care during an ambulatory procedure is safe completion of the procedure with minimal disruption of the patient's physiologic functions and comfort levels so that the patient may be returned to his or her home the same day. With that goal in mind, this chapter reviews preparation of the environment for the patient, describes care of the patient during the procedure, and lists specific nursing strategies you can employ when caring for an ambulatory patient during a procedure. Competent and compassionate care of the ambulatory patient during a procedure can facilitate safe completion of the procedure, minimize the patient's discomfort, and enhance the probability of a good outcome. This chapter focuses on general care of the ambulatory patient during surgery. Chapter 13 discusses care of the patient during special diagnostic and therapeutic procedures; Chapter 12 addresses concerns specific to the surgical specialties. A summary and a review of the critical concepts presented close the chapter.

## PREPARING THE ENVIRONMENT

Meticulous attention to preparation of the environment for the patient will not only facilitate safe and timely performance of the procedure, but will increase patient comfort and may avert disaster. This section summarizes general nursing actions that prepare the environment for the ambulatory patient.

## The Procedure Suite

Preparing a surgery suite or procedure room for patient care involves a knowledge of asepsis, the procedure itself, the surgeon's and anesthetist's preferences, and the patient's condition. Trained personnel with skills to meet these needs are usually assigned to the procedure. For ambulatory surgery, this personnel team may include a circulating nurse, a scrub nurse or surgical technician, the surgeon, and an anesthetist. When each performs his or her duties in a skilled and professional manner, patient safety and comfort are enhanced.

- Asepsis: Whenever surgery is performed, asepsis must be maintained to reduce the risk of microbial contamination that could harm the patient. Surgical nursing textbooks describe aseptic techniques in detail and you should refer to one of these resources for detailed information on this essential knowledge. Asepsis is also enhanced by room design, humidity, temperature, air flow, sterilization procedures, and surgical apparel.

- Temperature: Dressed in gowns and laboring under bright lights, surgical teams often request that the room temperature be lowered well into the sixty-degree range. This enhances their comfort and reduces the opportunity for microbial growth, but can lead to serious hypothermia in the patient. The anesthetist and circulating nurse can combat this by applying warming devices to the patient. These devices include: heat and moisture exchangers (a small inexpensive disposable device placed in the anesthesia breathing circuit), a humidifier placed into the anesthesia circuit, warming blankets that circulate warm air over the patient or warm water in coils under the patient, and heat retaining foil blankets and caps. The anesthetist may place clear plastic bags (discarded from equipment opened for the case) over and around the anesthetized patient's arms, legs and head to reduce heat loss. Another method to prevent hypothermia is warming intravenous fluids with devices specifically designed for that purpose. If the patient's temperature drops, the surgeon should be informed in hopes that in the patient's interest a compromise can be reached on the room temperature.

- Equipment: Prior to beginning any procedure the nurse should check equipment used in the surgery suite for proper functioning, because malfunctioning electrical and pneumatic equipment may cause patient and staff injury. Equipment should be inspected at regular intervals; the nurse should check to insure that such inspections have been completed. Any question about equipment functioning must be resolved before the equipment is used on the patient, because patient injury could result. Lasers are in common use in ambulatory patient care. Use of this powerful equipment requires special training, certification, and eye protection for both the staff and patient. Every day locate, for your reference, the crash code cart and the malignant hyperthermia supplies (if general anesthesia is administered in your area). The stress of a patient emergency will prove challenging enough without having to waste precious moments frantically searching for this equipment.

- Supplies: Familiarity with the surgeon's preferences and the procedure facilitates gathering the necessary supplies for the procedure. Most institutions keep records of a surgeon's preferences either on special cards or the computer. Having all necessary supplies in the suite can reduce the time needed to complete the procedure. Counting the supplies used in the wound, such as sponges and needles, is one way to insure that nothing is left behind in the patient. It is usually

# CHAPTER 8 —
# NURSING CARE OF THE PATIENT DURING THE PROCEDURE

the nurse's responsibility to check and recheck before signing off that the counts are correct.

## Ambience

Preparing the environment for the patient would be incomplete without attention to the ambience or mood of the suite. Loud music, raucous laughter, inappropriate or boisterous conversations, and inattention to the patient may all act to increase the patient's anxiety and reduce the patient's confidence in the professional competency of the staff. What is common and routine to the staff in the suite is seldom common or ordinary to the ambulatory patient. Every patient should feel as if he or she is the focus of the staff's attention and the most important person in the room at that time. Respectful professional care is a fundamental patient right; breaching this principle may result in litigation, adverse publicity, and public portrayal of the staff in a negative light (Murphy, 1993).

# CARING FOR THE PATIENT

In ambulatory surgery, the nurse caring for the patient during the procedure usually differs from the nurse who prepares the patient for the procedure. Communication of information is therefore essential as the patient is transferred to the operating room. The nursing process begun in the preparatory phase should be continued on into this procedure phase; referring to the initial nursing diagnoses will help the receiving nurse continue the care plan. While specific nursing strategies you can use when caring for the patient during the procedure are discussed in the next section, below you will find general guidelines for that care. At this point, nursing care is directed toward the goal of a safe outcome for the procedure while minimizing patient discomfort and distress.

## Admission

As the patient arrives in the operating room (OR) or procedure room, the nurse should greet the patient, then check and double-check that this is the right patient for the right procedure on the right part of the body at the right time in the right place by the right surgeon. Verify this not only against the chart but confirm this verbally with the patient as well. The chart should be reviewed; common information you should confirm includes the: history and physical, consent for the procedure, results of laboratory and diagnostic reports, preanesthesia evaluation if indicated, allergies, and NPO status. Follow your institution's specific policies when admitting the patient to the procedure room, but be aware that placing a patient on the OR table before the surgeon is present in the OR can put you in an awkward position if the surgeon is delayed whether in traffic or with another patient. Anesthesia is generally not administered until the surgeon is present, for the same reason.

## Assessment

After receiving report from the nurse who prepared the patient, you should be aware of the nursing diagnoses, the patient's needs, and expected outcomes. Review the diagnoses and briefly assess your patient so you can determine priorities. For example, reducing anxiety will clearly be a priority if your patient begins crying or trembling upon entrance to the procedure room. You may also identify other needs such as ineffective thermoregulation if your patient complains of feeling cold.

## Positioning

The patient should be as comfortable as possible on the procedure table in order to prevent injury. If general anesthesia is planned, the patient will lie supine for induction. In the event regional anesthesia is planned, the anesthetist will direct positioning of the patient. The nurse should remain at the bedside continuously until the patient is secured in the proper position, otherwise the patient might fall. In a few cases, the patient may be sedated or anesthetized on the stretcher, and then turned prone to the procedure table. This requires an adequate number of people to prevent injury to the patient or staff during the positioning maneuver. Surgical nursing textbooks usually have detailed chapters on positioning the patient in surgery; refer to one of these resources for further information.

## Monitoring

Monitors yield data which the anesthetist, nurse, or surgeon consider when caring for the patient. Monitors are devices that can fail or yield false data; you should not be lulled into a sense of security by relying exclusively on monitoring equipment. The monitors needed on a case vary according to the type of case and the patient's condition, but as a minimum generally include pulse oximetry, blood pressure, and electrocardiogram. Monitors can enhance patient safety, but the primary monitor of the patient in surgery is the anesthetist. In the absence of an anesthetist, the nurse usually assumes this function. Chapter 5, General Anesthesia, describes different monitors.

## Preparing the site

The operative site is cleansed and prepared after taking into consideration the surgeon's protocol, the facility's standards, the patient's condition, and the planned procedure. The purpose of cleansing the site is to reduce microorganisms; this will reduce the potential for infection. Surgical nursing textbooks describe site preparation in detail along with the principles involved if you need more information. Strict attention to proper site preparation can enhance the probability of achieving the expected outcome of the surgery. Infection rates are monitored by many facilities as a quality care indicator. Attend to the patient's dignity and privacy during this preparation; avoid exposing the patient unnecessarily.

## Documentation

Most facilities have operative record forms that the nurse completes on each patient. Many records are designed to expedite this process with simple check-off boxes. In any case, documentation should reflect the care given the patient, any deviations or complications, interventions, and outcomes. Perioperative documentation is essential in providing goal-directed care and evaluating the patient's response to care before, during, and after surgical intervention. Documentation of information about the patient's perioperative care provides an accurate picture of the phases and results of the care that has been delivered (AORN J., 1991). See Appendix B for AORN's Recommended Practices on Documentation of Perioperative Nursing Care.

When the nurse is responsible for administering sedation and monitoring the patient, those actions should be consistent with your facility's guidelines, your training and your skills, and within the scope of your license to practice nursing. Appendix B includes AORN's Recommended Practices on Monitoring the Patient Receiving IV Conscious Sedation.

Fig. 8-1, Universal Sedation Form, is an example of a record developed for use when nurses and others are administering sedation for special procedures.

## Family and support person's care

The support person or family who may be accompanying the patient should know where to wait for the patient and in general how long it will be before the patient is returned to them or they are informed of the patient's condition. A comfortable and quiet place for them to wait should be provided. Refreshments, diversions such as magazines and television, and telephones should be available. Many surgical facilities prefer that the family or support person not leave the facility, because of the possbility of an emergency or complication. The circulating nurse often notifies the support person or family once the

# CHAPTER 8 —
## NURSING CARE OF THE PATIENT DURING THE PROCEDURE

**Figure 8-1.** Universal Sedation Form.

**UNIVERSAL SEDATION POLICY**
**St. Francis Hospital**

1. The manufacturer's suggested guidelines of administration will be posted and made available for physician and staff referral.

2. Patients receiving I.V. sedation (i.e. VERSED, VALIUM, DEMEROL, etc.) must have baseline vital signs charted <u>prior to any sedation.</u>

3. All medications used will be charted on the <u>universal sedation form</u> including the amount, time given, type and route.

4. Patients will be monitored by pulse oximeter and/or appropriate monitoring equipment prior, during and post procedure. When the pulse oximeter is applied, the Sa $O_2$ % and the pulse rate will be documented on the chart. The alarm will be set routinely at 100% for high and 90% for low.

5. Vital signs will be monitored and charted <u>during, immediately following procedure and every 10 minutes X2</u> before the patient is released from the procedure area. If the vital signs are NOT within normal limits, they should be taken every 5 minutes until stable.

6. Patients may be released and pulse oximeter removed when they have met the routine discharge criteria of following simple commands with <u>erect</u> muscle tone, lifting head for 3 seconds and vital signs being stable.

7. If the patient's condition is not stable, their physician will be notified and if he/she desires, arrangements will be made with the recovery room to monitor the patient until stable.

8. If the patient remains unstable, the physician will decide when and where to release the patient. A nurse from the appropriate department will accompany the patient to the recovery room, outpatient department or patient's room. The receiving department will be given a verbal and written report.

9. Should the patient develop critical respiratory depression, refer to the CODE PURPLE Policy and Procedure.

   CODE PURPLE: Should a patient develop critical respiratory depression, a CODE PURPLE will be called by either the physician or representative departmental nurse. A CODE PURPLE will call a Respiratory Therapist to the department for immediate ambu of the patient, as well as a CRNA for possible intubation.

10. If VERSED is being administered, dosages will be 2 mg. with 2 minute intervals between dosing. 1 mg. test dosage will be done on patients age 65 years or older prior to proceeding with procedure using ½ doses.

01/30/90; Approved Med.Exec. Comm. 02/23/90

**Figure 8-1 (Cont.)** Universal Sedation Form. *Source:* St. Francis Hospital, Memphis, TN.

procedure is underway, and usually at about one hour intervals thereafter. The support person or family should know which facility employee they can turn to if they become concerned at other times. However, be certain that you do not give out information about the patient to anyone other than those designated by the patient, because this can breach confidentiality.

## Discharge from the procedure room

The nurse documents the patient's condition upon termination of the procedure and prepares the patient to return home or for transfer to a recovery area. Recovery from anesthesia is discussed in the following chapter. Any untoward events should be described and reported to the next caregiver; any medications administered by the nurse should be documented and reported. This will help the next nurse continue the care plan.

Transfer of the patient should be completed without delays in hallways or elevators. Also note that swiftly slinging patients off the procedure table and onto the stretcher can cause the patient pain and induce nausea or vomiting, as can rapid maneuvers around corners or spinning the stretcher 180-degrees in order to slip into a recovery room slot. These rapid motions should be avoided; when possible the patient may be allowed to move himself or herself to or from the stretcher in order to reduce nausea associated with motion sickness.

# NURSING STRATEGIES

The strategies for caring for an ambulatory patient during a procedure are complex and numerous; detailed information can be found in medical and surgical textbooks. Below however, are basic nursing strategies and the rationale behind each. These should prove helpful as you care for a patient during an ambulatory procedure. As always, your intervention should be within the scope of your institution's practice guidelines, consistent your state's Nurse Practice Act and your license, and commensurate with your skills and training.

- Introduce team members and their role to the patient upon entering the surgical suite. Even though personnel may be gowned and masked, such information accompanied by a greeting from the person can help reduce patient anxiety and increase patient confidence in the staff.

- Keep personnel not involved in the patient's care out of the surgical suite. This is important because it helps maintain confidentiality and a professional atmosphere, it protects the patient's privacy, and it reduces the chance of contamination of the room by outside air or microbes. Restricted access is absolutely essential during procedures where the patient may be conscious and exposed; to do otherwise may cause the patient embarrassment and increase anxiety.

- Treat the patient with respect and not as just another case to be done as quickly as possible. This is a fundamental patient right and it forms the foundation for positive professional care.

- Offer the patient simple explanations for the monitors and equipment used in the procedure. Explaining to the patient that the clip on the finger (pulse oximeter) lets the staff know that he or she is getting enough oxygen or that the cold pad on the leg is necessary because of the use of certain electrical equipment (cautery) can help decrease patient anxiety and increase patient confidence.

- Follow your institution's policy regarding the use of lasers. Lasers are powerful equipment capable of serious damage in the hands of the inexperienced or when certain protective measures are not taken.

- Expose only the area necessary when preparing the operative site; patient embarrassment, dismay, and chilling may result from unnecessary exposure.

- Consider placing a pillow or rolled blanket under the knees of the supine conscious patient during surgery; this will usually reduce lower back strain and enhance patient comfort. Elderly patients undergoing cataract surgery especially appreciate this.

- Investigate all patient complaints of discomfort during the procedure because injury may result when the staff ignores or discounts the patient's complaints.

- Restrict your conversation to positive or professional topics once the patient is in the operating room; refrain from complaining about being assigned to the case or grumbling about malfunctioning equipment. Such comments may stimulate fear, anxiety, and catecholamine release in the patient. The only thing the patient should hear is how important he or she is to the staff and how hard they are going to work in hopes of achieving a positive outcome.

- Address the adult patient by his or her name, such as Mr. or Mrs. Smith, not by familiar names such as "honey," "sweetie," or "grandpa." While you may feel quite close and nurturing to the patient as his or her nurse, the patient often does not share that bond with you. Patients may consider this imposed familiarity demeaning and it can reduce their confidence in your professionalism.

- Remember that while you may go to an ambulatory surgery facility everyday, your patient does not. Simple explanations and acknowledgement that some aspects of the experience can be frightening will help the patient feel more secure and less anxious.

- Note that sounds may be distorted to the patient who has received sedatives and other anesthetic agents. A quiet environment free of loud music, boisterous activity, and extraneous conversation can help reduce patient anxiety.

- Adhere to your facility's and the manufacturer's safety guidelines when using laser equipment, because serious patient or personnel injury could result from deviations from these standards.

- Keep the narcotic antagonist and benzodiazepine antagonist (naloxone or Narcan, and flumazenil or Romazicon) on hand whenever narcotics or benzodiazepine drugs such as morphine, fentanyl (Sublimaze), or midazolam (Versed) are used for sedation. Antagonists can reverse some or all of the effects of these drugs in the event that the patient becomes oversedated. These antagonists would ordinarily be administered by the physician or a member of the anesthesia team called to assist in this crisis.

- Don't administer drugs you are not familiar with, because patient injury and personal liability could result.

- Maintain voice contact with conscious patients who are covered by surgical drapes; leave at least one of the patient's hands exposed for observation of color and palpation of the pulse as necessary. This helps in your continuing assessment of the patient during the procedure.

- Don't rely completely on patient monitors to assess your patient because such reliance may lead to false conclusions. Monitors only display data; your brain must interpret and validate this information against the patient's condition.

- Use your nursing assessment skills to confirm information you derive from patient monitors. Remember that it is the patient's condition that is important, not his or her numbers. For example, a healthy young woman with a blood pressure (BP) of 86/50, resting quietly in the preop holding area, almost certainly requires no treatment for hypotension. But when a 58-year-old man with a history of coronary artery disease and preoperative BPs averaging 160/100 drops to a BP of 86/50 during surgery, further assessment and investigation are warranted.

- Be aware that human error occasionally results in a patient arriving for a procedure with a chart, orders, progress notes, diagnostic reports or other documents that are not theirs. This could have disastrous consequences if overlooked. Double-check the imprints on the chart and records and confirm the patient's name and doctor verbally with him or her; check this against the patient's ID band.

- Be aware that some plastic surgeons want to photograph or mark landmarks or planned incision lines on a patient before beginning surgery. Once sedation is administered the patient will be unable to stand and may have difficulty even in sitting, so you should know the surgeon's preferences before any sedation is given.

- Avoid placing the patient on the procedure table until the physician is in the facility. Otherwise, if the physician's arrival is delayed, the patient may have to anxiously lay in wait until his or her arrival. This usually causes patient discomfort, increases operating room fees, and may delay other cases.

- Note that many patients will want to see their doctor before induction of anesthesia; notify the physician and anesthetist if this is the case.

- Turn your attention to the patient during induction of anesthesia, because the anesthetist may require your assistance. Many patients also appreciate the reassuring presence of their nurse at the bedside at this time.

- Ask the anesthetist if you may simply hold the anesthesia mask directly over but not touching the patient's face if the patient expresses a fear of having the mask on his or her face while being prepared for induction of general anesthesia. Some patients feel as if they are suffocating when the mask is strapped to their face, and panic may ensue. If the anesthetist allows the nurse to simply hold the mask near the face so the patient can breathe the oxygen, it usually relieves this fear while still providing the patient with oxygen-rich air.

- Insure a quiet professional environment during induction of anesthesia because sounds may be magnified to the patient at this time and hearing is the last sense to go.

- Note that after induction of general anesthesia, surgery should not begin until the patient's airway is secured. Establishing an airway is always first priority in any patient care setting.

- Follow your institution's policy on counting needles and sponges used during surgery and the protocol for steps to be taken when counts are not reconciled; this will help insure patient safety.

- Note that laser vaporization of certain growths such as condyloma (genital warts) is believed to result in particles of those growths being released into the procedure room's air. Inhalation by attending personnel could be potentially harmful, so special filtration masks should be worn. Some professionals also use a device that vacuums these airborne particles as they are released.

- Remember that events not easily treated (such as operating on the wrong part of the body or a patient fall from the OR table) should be prevented.

- Monitor patient warming devices carefully, because serious patient injury can result from using such devices on unconscious patients or those with anesthetized areas of their body (as from regional anesthesia).

- Slipping the unconscious patient's arms or legs into clear plastic bags during surgery can help reduce heat loss but still allow visualization of the limb.

- Sandwich the patient between warmed blankets by laying one on the procedure table before moving the patient onto it and then placing another next to the skin. This can help reduce patient heat loss to the table and may increase patient comfort.

- Do not heat intravenous fluids or surgical solutions in devices not intended for that purpose, such as microwave ovens, because the resulting temperature is unpredictable and may cause patient injury. Heating such solutions also has the potential to change the composition of the solution or container.

- Never use equipment in the OR for a purpose other than that for which it was intended; doing otherwise could compromise patient care or cause injury to the patient or staff.

- Do not say anything during administration of a general anesthetic that you would not say if the patient was conscious, because intraoperative awareness is possible. Such comments can cause the patient distress and may result in professional liability and embarrassment.

- Act as the advocate when necessary for anesthetized patients who cannot speak for themselves. This helps insure that the patient's rights and dignity are preserved.

- Keep a small personal stereo headset (like a Sony Walkman) in the procedure room and offer to let the conscious or lightly sedated patient listen to music during the procedure if the anesthetist and surgeon agree. An assortment of pre-recorded cassettes in a variety of music should be on hand, because clear radio reception can sometimes be difficult to obtain inside the facility. Music can help reduce the patient's anxiety (Steelman, 1990), distract the patient during uncomfortable procedures, and diminish awareness of OR equipment such as drills and saws.

- Take care in discussing abnormal pathology reports in the presence of a sedated patient, because the patient may presume this information pertains to them when it may not.

- Be courteous and prompt in responding to the support person's or family member's request for information about the progress of the procedure, especially if the procedure has been delayed. This can help reduce their anxiety and increase their confidence and satisfaction in the facility.

- Insist that an adequate number of personnel be present when an anesthetized or sedated patient's position must be changed on the procedure table. Such patients are prone to falls and injury and the presence of a sufficient number of personnel will increase the probability of a safe position change.

- Do not disable alarms on equipment used in surgery; this could result in patient injury.

- Know in advance of need how to call for emergency teams. In the event of a patient crisis or

# CHAPTER 8 — NURSING CARE OF THE PATIENT DURING THE PROCEDURE

fire, seconds count and time spent looking up a number or searching for a fire alarm or extinguisher could result in serious harm or loss.

- Don't leave the anesthetist alone with an anesthetized patient, because an emergency could arise and he or she might be unable to secure help.

- Leave the safety restraint on the patient until the team is ready to transfer the patient from the procedure table to the stretcher. Without the restraint in place the patient may fall from the table.

- Remain close to the bedside during the patient's emergence from general anesthesia because this can be a hazardous phase and the anesthetist may require your assistance.

- Keep the procedure room door closed to reduce potential for entrance of outside air with possible microbes, and to protect patient privacy.

- Resolve doubts about asepsis in favor of the patient: if in doubt about whether sterile technique was broken, presume that it was. This will help reduce the chance for infection.

- Label all specimens exactly as instructed and follow protocol in transporting specimens. Losing or mislabeling a specimen could have disastrous consequences.

- Move the patiently gently after surgery because jostling and jerking can cause pain. Swift motions should also be avoided in patients prone to N & V, especially if associated with motion sickness.

- Determine in consultation with your facility's medical and nursing directors whether or not intravenous access should be established on patients coming to the OR for local anesthesia when anesthesia personnel will not be in attendance. While complications are rare, the development of a toxic reaction to the local anesthetic or a serious arrhythmia can be disastrous in a patient without an IV line.

- Have oxygen, suction, and manual resuscitation bag and mask available in the room when the patient is having local anesthesia in the absence of anesthesia personnel. In the event of an emergency, this will save precious time.

- Know in advance of need the location of the crash (code) cart and malignant hyperthermia supplies. This will save valuable time in the event of an emergency.

# SUMMARY

The goal of nursing care during a procedure is safe completion of the procedure with minimal disruption of the ambulatory patient's physiologic functions and comfort levels, so that the patient may be returned to his or her home the same day. This chapter reviewed preparation of the environment for the patient, described care of the patient during the procedure, and listed specific nursing strategies you can employ when caring for an ambulatory patient during a procedure.

# CRITICAL CONCEPTS

- Avoid errors. Check and double-check to make sure you have the right patient for the right procedure on the right part of the body at the right time in the right place by the right surgeon. Verify this not only against the chart but ask the patient as well.

- Treat patients with respect and dignity. This is a fundamental patient right that can also reduce the chance for professional embarrassment and litigation.

- Note that what is routine and commonplace to you as a healthcare professional is seldom routine to your patient. Focus your attention on the patient and offer reassurances and frequent simple explanations of activities and equipment.

- Meticulous preparation and scrupulous attention to asepsis will enhance the probability of a good outcome of the surgery for the patient.

- The nurse's actions during the procedure can mean the difference between a good outcome and bad outcome for the patient.

# EXAM QUESTIONS

## Chapter 8

Questions 45-49

45. A good method of warming the patient during surgery is:

    a. infusing microwave-heated intravenous fluids
    b. increasing the humidity in the room
    c. using cold irrigation solutions to stimulate shivering
    d. applying a patient warming blanket ✓

46. A common nursing diagnosis of the patient during surgery is:

    a. pain
    b. parenting alteration
    c. verbal communication impairment
    d. fear ✓

47. The basic monitors generally required during surgery include blood pressure, electrocardiogram, and:

    a. temperature
    b. foley catheter
    c. end-tidal $CO_2$
    d. pulse oximeter ✓

48. What should the nurse have available on the unit whenever narcotics are administered?

    a. propofol (Diprivan)
    b. sodium citrate (Bicitra)
    c. neostigmine (Prostigmin)
    d. naloxone (Narcan) ✓

49. It is best to maintain a professional atmosphere during surgery, even when general anesthesia is administered, because of possible:

    a. patient amnesia
    b. intraoperative awareness ✓
    c. postprocedure paralysis
    d. intraoperative hypotension

# CHAPTER 9

# NURSING CARE OF THE PATIENT AFTER THE PROCEDURE

## CHAPTER OBJECTIVE

After completing this chapter, you should be better prepared to care for your patient during the period of time immediately following an ambulatory procedure.

## LEARNING OBJECTIVES

After reading this chapter, you should be able to:

1. Identify nursing actions that enhance the comfort and safety of the patient recovering from anesthesia.

2. Select potential nursing diagnoses for the postanesthesia patient.

3. Differentiate among common complications that may arise during the immediate postanesthesia phase.

4. Indicate priorities in planning nursing care for the postanesthesia patient.

5. Identify ways in which the type of anesthetic administered will influence the nurse's plan of care for that patient.

6. Recognize the usual progression of recovery from general and regional anesthesia.

7. Recognize physiologic changes that may develop during recovery from general anesthesia.

## INTRODUCTION

This chapter focuses generally on the care of the ambulatory patient immediately after a procedure, but more specifically on the care of the postoperative patient. Reviewing the usual progression of recovery from anesthesia, this chapter describes general nursing care of the patient immediately after the procedure and lists specific nursing strategies you can employ when caring for the ambulatory patient. Common postoperative complaints of the ambulatory patient are addressed. A summary and a review of the critical concepts presented close the chapter. Nurses assigned to postanesthesia care units may want to review a postanesthesia nursing textbook because more detailed information can be found there.

## RECOVERY FROM ANESTHESIA

Despite the development of short-acting anesthetic agents, the effects of anesthesia are not simply terminated when the patient rolls out of the procedure room; these effects may continue for a period of several hours, especially if short-acting agents were not used or when some regional techniques such as epidurals are used. This places a tremendous amount of responsibility on the postanesthesia nurse, who must be prepared for the worst while striving for the best. Caring for the ambulatory patient necessitates some modifications in postanesthesia nursing care because the ambulatory patient is expected to leave the facility that day in a condition that the support person will be able to manage in the home. This means that another person, usually a non-professional, will be sharing responsibility for patient recovery.

Below you will find described the basics of recovery from general, regional and local anesthesia. This is not a complete discussion; you can find detailed information in a postanesthesia nursing textbook. This information is presented as an overview of the postanesthesia phase of ambulatory patient care. Don't forget that just as each patient is unique, recovery from anesthesia is a highly individualized process and may vary widely from one patient to another. Factors influencing recovery from anesthesia include the type of anesthesia administered, the length of the surgical procedure, and the patient's age and condition (Chitwood, 1992).

## General anesthesia

As discussed in Chapter 5, general anesthesia (GA) is usually induced with a combination of drugs and anesthetic agents that are inhaled and injected. The final phase of general anesthesia is emergence. Emergence begins in the operating room (OR) as the anesthetic agents are discontinued and reversal agents are administered as needed. Emergence continues in the postanesthesia care unit (PACU) under the care of the nurse. The risk of complications from anesthesia persists until emergence is complete. As the patient drifts back up into consciousness there may be some confusion or disorientation; reassuring and orienting the patient to time and place usually relieves it. Ambulatory anesthesia has been revolutionized by the development of short-acting intravenous agents such as propofol (Diprivan) and inhalation agents such as desflurane (Suprane). The effects of these anesthetic agents are rapidly terminated so emergence is swift; patients are often alert enough to move themselves from the operating room (OR) table and frequently are able to state their needs for warmth, po liquids, or pain medicine immediately upon arrival in the PACU.

## Regional anesthesia

Recovery from regional anesthesia may be nearly complete upon admission to the PACU in some cases, as with an intravenous regional technique. In other cases, such as spinal anesthesia, more prolonged effects may result. Do not overlook the effects of sedatives and narcotics commonly administered to enhance patient comfort during regional anesthesia; these also lead to somnolence. Patients will often voice concern about the return of sensation and function to the anesthetized area; nurses should patiently hear these concerns and then reassure the patient that recovery is generally uneventful.

- **Spinal anesthesia:** Recovery from spinal anesthesia may take several hours; this can distress patients who may become concerned that permanent paralysis has developed. Reassurance usually allays this fear. Patients who have had spinal anesthesia may be asked to remain flat to reduce the potential for a spinal headache (see Chapter 6, Regional Anesthesia); check the facility or anesthetist's policy for guidance.

- **Epidural anesthesia:** Unless the dura was inadvertently punctured during placement of the epidural anesthetic (see Chapter 6), there will be no need for the patient to lie flat. Recovery may again take several hours and reassurance may be necessary for the concerned patient. Sometimes a small amount of an opioid analgesic such as

# CHAPTER 9 —
## NURSING CARE OF THE PATIENT AFTER THE PROCEDURE

morphine or fentanyl (Sublimaze) is injected through the epidural catheter for postoperative pain control.

- Intravenous regional anesthesia: Intravenous regional anesthesia is administered by filling the veins of the lower part of the extremity with a local anesthetic (LA) such as xylocaine (see Chapter 6). A tourniquet restricts the LA to the extremity; this tourniquet is released when the surgery is completed. The LA then flows into the bloodstream, but its potency is sharply reduced due to the body's metabolism. Nevertheless, this LA has the potential to cause a seizure or other stimulation of the central nervous system. This may develop in the OR or the PACU.

- Nerve blocks: Sensorimotor function returns gradually after a nerve block; the nurse's major focus is to protect the extremity until function and sensation return. For example, the patient will be unaware that his fingers are pinched in the stretcher railing if the extremity is anesthetized, so the nurse must be vigilant for him or her until sensation returns.

### Local anesthesia

Because complications from local anesthetics are rare but most likely to be manifested soon after injection, patients who had a procedure under local anesthesia without any sedation often bypass Phase 1 of the recovery process and move straight into the discharge phase. If the patient received any sedation though, he or she will need to be assessed for recovery from those effects before transfer.

# AFTER THE PROCEDURE

The goal of nursing care immediately after an ambulatory procedure is to restore the patient to at least his or her previous level of wellness through an uneventful recovery, so the patient can return home that same day. Postanesthesia nurses who care for patients during their recovery from anesthesia must possess a broad knowledge of the different types of anesthetics and the effects on the patient. There are excellent postanesthesia nursing care textbooks available with this information; this section only serves as an overview. Table 9-1 reveals common nursing diagnoses for patients recovering from anesthesia.

After ambulatory surgery, postanesthesia care usually involves a two-step plan of care: the first phase encompasses the acute phase of recovery from anesthesia, the second phase prepares the patient for discharge to home. Phase 1 generally takes place in a specially designated area such as a postanesthesia unit (PACU) and encompasses the period of time of emergence from anesthesia until the patient is stable and awake. After phase 1, in some facilities the patient is transferred to another area of the facility that has a more casual atmosphere. This may be a private room or a single large room for several patients. The support person or family are often a part of this phase, as the patient gradually sits up in a reclining chair and begins to take nourishment. The patient will also attempt to void and ambulate. In some facilities phase 1 and 2 both take place in the PACU. When the patient meets criteria, he or she is usually assisted with dressing, given discharge instructions, and escorted to waiting transportation. Phase 2 is discussed in greater detail in the next chapter, Nursing Care of the Patient During the Discharge Phase. This chapter focuses on the first phase of recovery. Wherever the patient's postprocedure care takes

## Table 9-1
## Potential Nursing Diagnoses for Patients Recovering from Anesthesia

| Nursing Diagnosis | Nursing Intervention |
| --- | --- |
| Anxiety related to situational crisis (surgery) | Give clear concise explanations; offer verbal reassurance; stay with patient who exhibits severe anxiety; request the anesthetist evaluate the patient for possible administration of a tranquilizer if necessary. |
| Airway clearance, ineffective, related to presence of tracheobronchial obstruction or secretions, or to fatigue (from neuromuscular blockade) | Have suction available at bedside in OR and PACU; suction patient prn to keep airway clear; administer oxygen as ordered; do not extubate patient until all parameters established by your institution have been met; ask anesthetist to evaluate a patient who appears to be weak with residual neuromuscular blockade; position unconscious patient on side to reduce chance of tongue obstructing airway; prepare for reintubation in the patient who experiences a laryngospasm that is not relieved by suctioning, jaw lift, and positive pressure oxygen by mask; know the location of emergency airway equipment; if in doubt about the patient's respiratory status, ask anesthetist to evaluate patient. |
| Fluid volume deficit, potential, related to active loss | Monitor vital signs as indicated postoperatively; administer IV fluids as ordered; assess skin turgor and urine output; consult with surgeon and anesthetist as indicated by the patient's condition; administer antiemetics as ordered to halt fluid loss by vomiting. |
| Pain related to physical agent (surgery) | Assess patient's pain and administer analgesics as prescribed; perform comfort measures such as repositioning; manipulate the environment to promote uninterrupted rest; apply heat or cold as ordered to minimize or relieve pain. |
| Sensory or perceptual alteration related to recovery from anesthetic agents | Reorient patient to present: call by name, tell patient your name, orient to environment; reduce excessive noise and lights; explain procedures, tests, equipment, and unusual sounds; help patient interpret environment by saying "This is the Recovery Room...I am your nurse...your operation is over...that sound you hear is the heart rhythm monitor...." |
| Thermoregulation, ineffective related to cold environ. during surgery/anesthesia | Monitor body temperature during and after surgery; apply warm blankets or warming devices and monitor their use and the patient's reaction carefully; replace wet linens or gowns with clean, warm, and dry ones; place warm blankets next to patient's skin and cover with additional blankets. |
| Aspiration, potential, related to surgery and anesthesia | Position unconscious patient on side to decrease risk of aspiration; do not offer liquids until the patient is fully awake, then offer moistened cloth first. Do not give patient anything by mouth until it has been determined that he or she is stable and a return to surgery is unlikely. |

*Please note this is a sample of potential nursing diagnoses and is not presented as, nor intended to be, a complete care plan for the recovering patient. More complete information can be found in a medical surgical nursing course and textbook.*

Adapted from: *Nursing Diagnosis Reference Manual* by Sheila Sparks and Cynthia M. Taylor, Springhouse Corporation, 1991.

place, the patient and family are always entitled to privacy and dignity when receiving that care.

Because disasters are easier to prevent than to treat, the PACU nurse should be well prepared for potential complications. This also makes routine care easier and more relaxed. Immediately on hand for the patient's arrival in the PACU should be functional suction tubing with an assortment of catheters, an oxygen source with mask or endotracheal tube adaptor, and syringes. Emergency drugs and supplies should be within the PACU and immediately available, as should a manual resuscitation bag (Ambu bag) in case manual ventilation of the patient becomes necessary. Communication of information is essential as care of the patient is handed over to the PACU nurse. The nursing process begun in the preparatory phase should be continued on into the recovery phase; referring to the initial nursing diagnoses will help the PACU nurse continue the care plan. While specific nursing strategies you can use when caring for the postprocedure patient are discussed in the next section, below you will find general guidelines for that care and common complications you might encounter.

## Admission to the PACU

Priorities in postanesthesia care remain the same, regardless of whether the patient is ambulatory or inpatient: first establish that the airway, breathing and circulation (ABC) are adequate. So, as the patient arrives in the PACU, the nurse should immediately assess the ABCs. This is done even while receiving a verbal report from the anesthetist regarding the procedure, type of anesthesia, any complications, medication administered, and the patient's significant medical history including allergies. After receiving report from the OR nurse or the anesthetist, you should be aware of the nursing diagnoses and expected outcomes.

- Airway and breathing: Nothing supersedes the priority of ascertaining that the patient's airway is patent and ventilation is adequate. This can be verified by feeling for air movement from the patient's nose and mouth, observing chest excursions, auscultating breath sounds, and pulse oximetry. In the event the airway is not patent or air exchange is not adequate, immediate intervention to establish an airway is essential. Figure 9-1 depicts methods of maintaining a patent airway.

- Circulation: A patent airway with adequate ventilation is the first priority; establishing that circulation is adequate follows. Circulation is evaluated by reviewing cardiac activity on an electrocardiogram display, auscultating heart sounds, palpating pulses, measuring blood pressure, and applying a pulse oximeter. Blood pressure swings are not unusual in postanesthesia patients. Hypotension may be the result of volume loss in surgery or the effects of anesthesia; hypertension may result from postoperative pain and may develop during emergence, especially if an endotracheal tube is acting as a noxious stimulus to the patient.

## Complications

After the ABCs, the nurse turns his or her attention to other patient needs identified through nursing diagnoses. Chapter 14 discusses common serious complications; below is a brief discussion of concerns that may disrupt a smooth recovery. Note that complications from regional and local anesthesia are generally manifested in the OR.

- Pain: Ambulatory patients have the same rights to analgesia as do inpatients, but a balance must be struck between relieving pain and not oversedating the patient or prolonging his or her stay in the ambulatory unit. Non-steroidal anti-inflammatory agents are filling this need because of their non-sedating analgesic action. Ketorolac (Toradol) is one of these agents that is proving useful in this area. Some surgeons will instill or

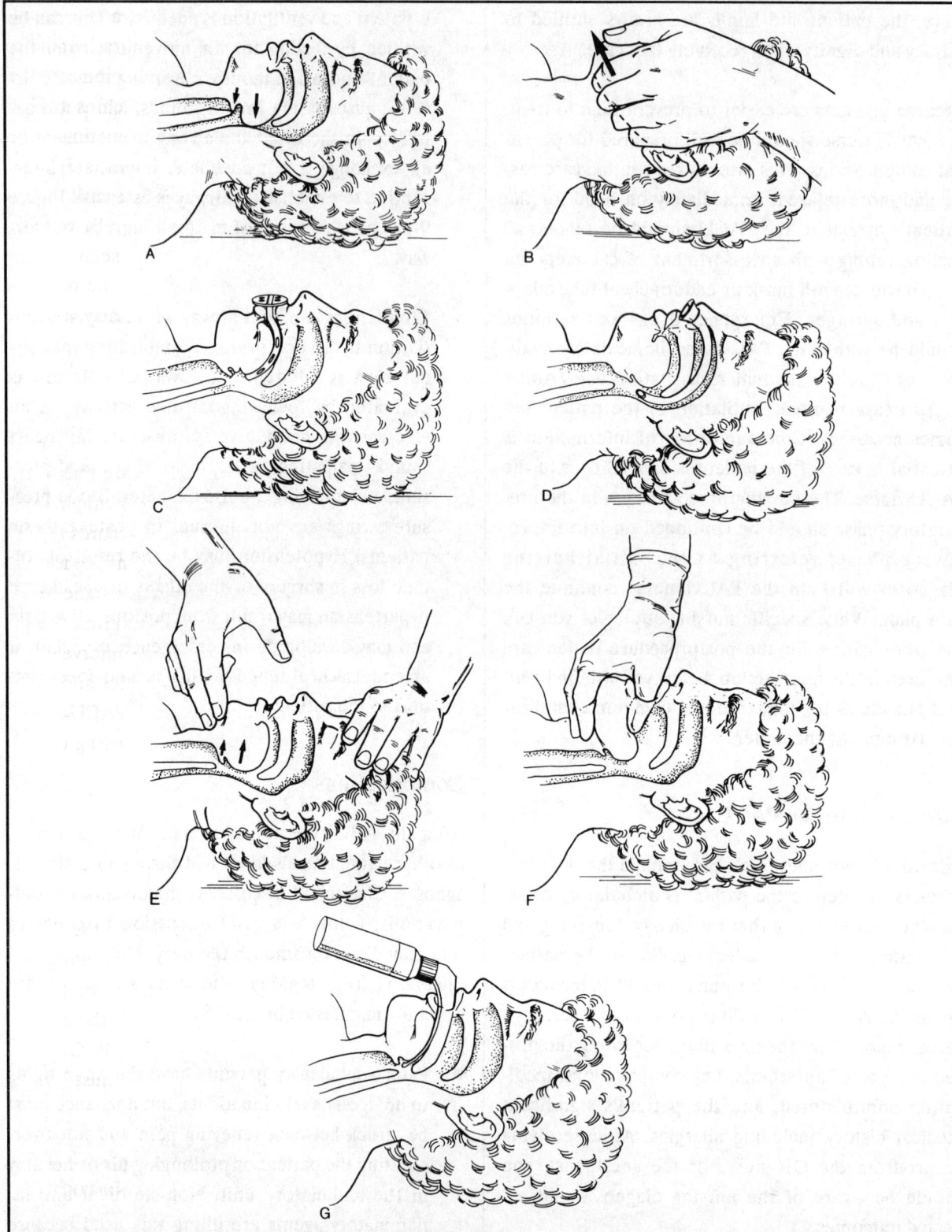

**Figure 9-1.** Maintaining the patient airway. (A) Obstructed airway (tongue against pharynx); (B) Manual jaw extension/jaw thrust (anterior placement); (C) Insertion of oral airway; (D) insertion of nasal airway; (E) Head tilt; (F) Manual tongue extension; (G) intubation.

*Source:* Burden, N. (1993) Ambulatory Surgical Nursing, W. B. Saunders Company.

infiltrate local anesthetic solutions into the wound or incision; this produces analgesia into the postoperative period. Unrelieved pain can lead to hypertension. See Fig. 9-2, Preventing and Relieving Postop Pain, for more on clinical pain management strategies. Fig. 9-3, Pain Treatment Flow Chart, guides you through the maze of managing postoperative pain.

- Nausea & Vomiting (N & V): One of the most common concerns and complaints of the ambulatory surgical patient is N & V. New anesthetic agents reduce the incidence of N & V postoperatively, but this will probably never be eradicated. Some types of surgeries are simply associated with a higher incidence of N & V. A small amount of droperidol (Inapsine) administered just before induction of anesthesia seems to be an effective prophylactic in many patients. Other patients, especially those prone to motion sickness, find relief with transdermal scopolamine patches (Trans-derm Scop), but this must be applied at least fours hours before surgery, and preferably the night before surgery. In other patients, administration of metoclopramide (Reglan) will hasten emptying of the stomach and reduce vomiting. A new antinauseant, ondansetron (Zofran) was recently introduced; it is quite expensive but may prove effective when other methods have failed.

- Hypothermia: Hypothermia is common in patients undergoing surgery and GA; recovery is often prolonged in the cold patient because of the lowered metabolism. Fortunately, new methods are reducing the incidence of hypothermia. Patient warming systems utilizing disposable air-filled blankets are quite effective at reducing heat loss during ambulatory surgery. Warm blankets and warming lights can also help alleviate hypothermia. Note that shivering is common during emergence from inhalation anesthesia; the etiology is unknown and this shivering may not always be the result of patient chilling.

- Emergence delirium: Occasionally a patient will become agitated, combative, and thrash about in the bed after GA. This is more common after administration of certain drugs such as scopolamine. Emergence delirium is sometimes successfully treated with physostigmine (Antilirium). Protecting the patient until the delirium passes is essential and generally requires several people. Note that what seems to be emergence delirium can simply be the result of unrelieved pain; anxious patients may also exhibit similar signs.

## Documentation

Because the patient seldom spends more than a few hours at most in the PACU, adequate documentation of care can be difficult. Many PACU records are designed to expedite this process with simple check-off boxes. However, documentation of postanesthesia care should genuinely reflect the care given the patient, any deviations or complications, interventions, and outcomes. Documenting the complex and highly skilled professional care given in the PACU should incorporate the nursing process and nursing diagnoses (Gay, 1990).

## Family and support person's care

The support person or family involved in the patient's aftercare is often reunited with the patient in the PACU or phase 2 area. They will require support and teaching as they prepare to assume responsibility for the patient at home. When the support person is allowed into the immediate PACU area, other patients' identities and privacy must still be maintained.

## Discharge from the postanesthesia room

Most ambulatory facilities have a protocol or set of guidelines for discharging the patient to phase 2 or to home. This may involve a scoring system that evaluates the patient's level of alertness, ability to move,

1. *Promise patients attentive analgesic care.* Patients should be informed before surgery, verbally and in printed format, that effective pain relief is an important part of their treatment, that talking about unrelieved pain is essential, and that health professionals will respond quickly to their reports of pain. It should be made clear to patients and families, however, that the total absence of any postoperative discomfort is normally not a realistic or even a desirable goal.

2. *Chart and display assessment of pain and relief.* A simple assessment of pain intensity and pain relief should be recorded on the bedside vital sign chart or a similar record that encourages easy, regular review by members of the health care team and is incorporated in the patient's permanent record. The intensity of pain should be assessed and documented at regular intervals (depending on the severity of pain) and with each new report of pain. The degree of pain relief should be determined after each pain management intervention, once a sufficient time has elapsed for the treatment to reach peak effect. A simple, valid measure of intensity and relief should be selected by each clinical unit. For children, age-appropriate measures should be used.

3. *Define pain and relief levels to trigger a review.* Each institution should identify pain intensity and pain relief levels that will elicit a review of the current pain therapy, documentation of the proposed modifications in treatment, and subsequent review of its efficacy. This process of treatment review and follow up should include participation by physicians and nurses involved in the patient's care.

4. *Survey patient satisfaction.* At regular intervals defined by the clinical unit and quality assurance committee, each clinical unit should assess a randomly selected sample of patients who have had surgery within 72 hours. Patients should be asked their current pain intensity, the worst pain intensity in the past 24 hours, the degree of relief obtained from pain management interventions, satisfaction with relief, and their satisfaction with the staff's responsiveness.

5. *Analgesic drug treatment should comply with several basic principles:*
   a. *Non-opioid "peripherally acting" analgesics.* Unless contraindicated, every patient should receive an around-the-clock postoperative regimen of an NSAID. For patients unable to take medications by mouth, it may be necessary to use the parenteral or rectal route.
   b. *Opioid analgesics.* Analgesic orders should allow for the great variation in individual opioid requirements, including a regularly scheduled dose and "rescue" doses for instances in which the usual regimen is insufficient.

6. *Specialized analgesic technologies,* including systemic or intraspinal, continuous or intermittent opioid administration or patient controlled dosing, local anesthetic infusion, and inhalational analgesia (e.g., nitrous oxide) should be governed by policies and standard procedures that define the acceptable level of patient monitoring and appropriate roles and limits of practice for all groups of health care providers involved. The policy should include definitions of physician and nurse accountability, physician and nurse responsibility to the patient, and the role of pharmacy.

**Figure 9–2.** Preventing and Relieving Postoperative Pain.

> 7. *Nonpharmacological interventions:* Cognitive and behaviorally based interventions include a number of methods to help patients understand more about their pain and to take an active part in its assessment and control. These interventions are intended to supplement, not replace, pharmacological interventions. Staff should give patients information about these interventions and support patients in using them.
>
> 8. *Monitor the efficacy of pain treatment:* Periodically review pain treatment procedures as defined in summary recommendations 1–4 above, using the institution's quality assurance procedures.
>
> **Figure 9–2 (cont.).** Preventing and Relieving Postoperative Pain.
> Source: Acute Pain Management Guideline panel. *Acute Pain Management: Operative or Medical Procedures and Trauma. Clinical Practice Guideline.* U.S. Department of Health and Human Services. Feb. 1992.

respirations, BP, color, fluid intake, and voiding. Discharge of the patient from the facility is discussed in Chapter 10.

# NURSING STRATEGIES

The strategies for caring for an ambulatory patient after surgery or a special procedure are complex and numerous; detailed information can be found in medical and surgical textbooks. Below however, are basic nursing strategies and the rationale behind each. These should prove helpful as you care for a patient after an ambulatory procedure. As always, your intervention should be within the scope of your institution's practice guidelines, consistent your state's Nurse Practice Act and your license, and commensurate with your skills and training.

- Introduce yourself and state your role to the conscious patient when he or she comes into your care in the PACU. This information accompanied by your greeting can help reduce patient anxiety and increase confidence in the staff.

- Offer the patient simple explanations for what you are doing. Explanations can help decrease patient anxiety and increase patient confidence.

- Orient and reassure the emerging patient frequently by repeating quietly such things as: "This is the recovery room...I am your nurse...you are just waking up...your surgery is over and everything went well...that sound you hear is the heart monitor; your heart and your blood pressure are fine and you are in good condition...." These explanations help reduce patient anxiety and may hasten orientation to the surroundings.

- Pull the drapes around the patient before you expose him or her to check the operative site. Expose only the area necessary; patient embarrassment, dismay, and chilling may result from unnecessary exposure.

- Check to insure that you have functioning suction and oxygen at patient care sites in the PACU and that appropriate supplies such as syringes, emesis basins, and towels are available. Leaving an arriving patient's bedside to search for basic and essential patient care supplies or to replace non-functioning equipment costs time and could impair patient care.

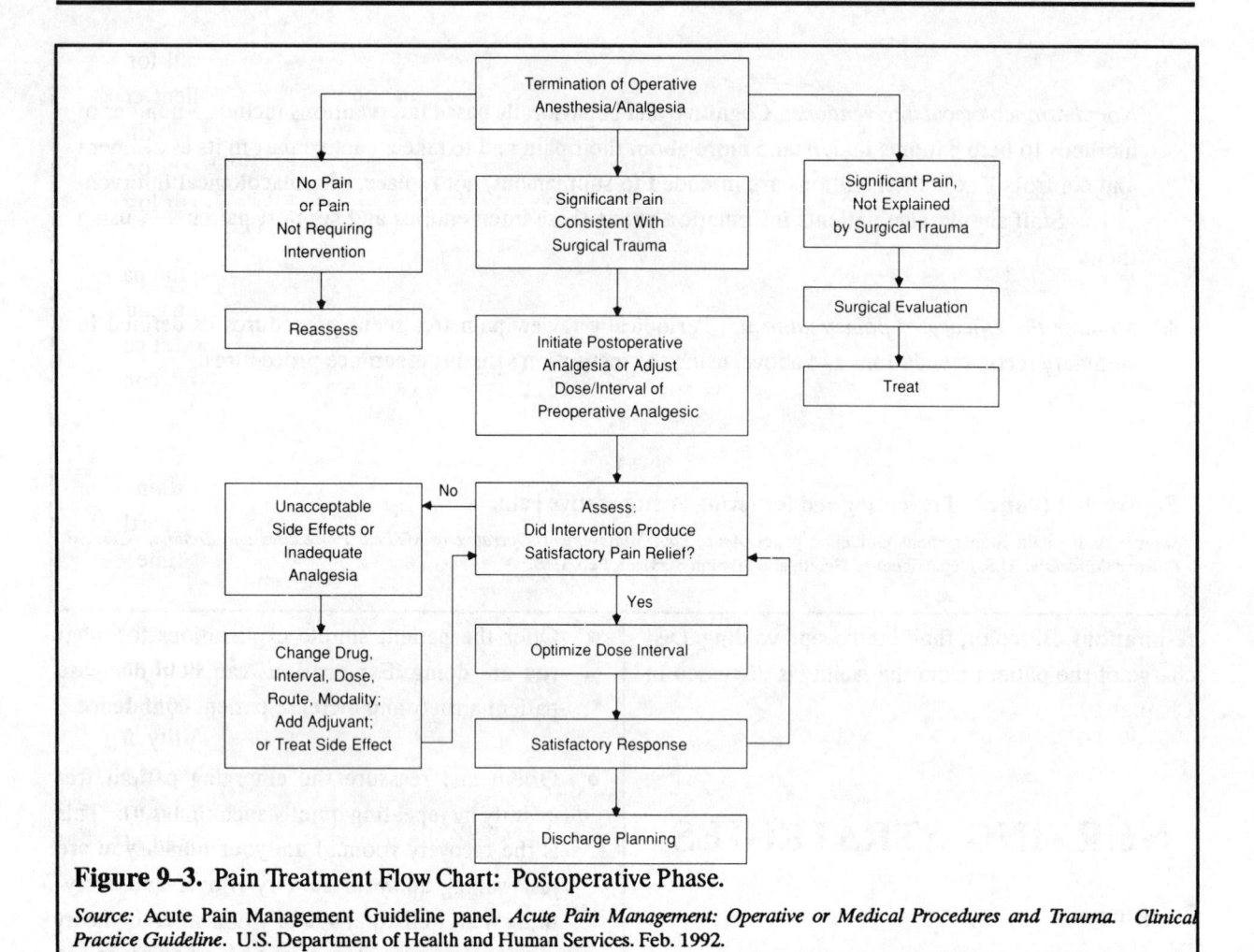

**Figure 9–3.** Pain Treatment Flow Chart: Postoperative Phase.

*Source:* Acute Pain Management Guideline panel. *Acute Pain Management: Operative or Medical Procedures and Trauma. Clinical Practice Guideline.* U.S. Department of Health and Human Services. Feb. 1992.

- Never leave the drapes pulled around an emerging or unconscious patient, because you will not be able to assess the patient's condition. Tragedy can occur in just a matter of minutes in an unattended and unseen patient.

- Note that sounds may be distorted to the patient as he or she recovers from general anesthesia. A quiet environment free of loud music, boisterous activity, and extraneous conversation can help facilitate a smooth emergence.

- Insure a quiet professional environment during recovery from anesthesia because sounds may be magnified to the patient during emergence and hearing is the first sense to return.

- Remember that events not easily treated (such as the patient falling from the stretcher in the PACU) should be prevented.

- Monitor patient warming devices carefully, because serious patient injury can result from improperly using such devices on sedated or unconscious patients.

- Place comfortably warm blankets directly against the patient's skin and then cover with another blanket to trap the warmth. Do this discreetly so as to protect the patient's privacy. This can help maintain the patient's core temperature and usually increases the patient's comfort.

- Maintain intravenous access until recovery from anesthesia is complete, because complications

# CHAPTER 9 —
## NURSING CARE OF THE PATIENT AFTER THE PROCEDURE

could still arise, or intravenous fluid may be necessary to combat dehydration if vomiting develops.

- Do not say anything around an emerging or drowsy patient that you would not say if the patient was awake, because hearing is the first sense to return. Inappropriate comments can cause the patient distress and may result in professional liability and embarrassment.

- Take care in discussing abnormal pathology reports in the presence of recovering patients, because patients or their support person may presume this information pertains to the patient and be alarmed or distressed. This can also violate the confidentiality of the patient the report does refer to.

- Do not slap a patient in an effort to hasten arousal from anesthesia. Doing so indicates disregard for the patient's dignity and rights, is usually ineffective, and may be considered inappropriate professional conduct. Shouting is generally ineffective and unnecessary and may serve only to distress the emerging patient.

- Offer cold carbonated soft drinks such as colas if the physician's orders and the patient's medical condition allows it. These cold drinks seem to reduce nausea and the headache that many patients develop from missing their morning coffee.

- Apply cold wet towels to the face, and mop around the neck of the patient who complains of nausea; exchange for more cold towels and continue until nausea subsides, usually in a few minutes. This often reduces the unpleasant sensation of nausea. Notify the physician or follow facility protocol if the nausea does not subside.

- Know in advance of need how to call for emergency teams. In the event of a patient crisis or fire, seconds count and time spent looking up a number or searching for a fire alarm or extinguisher could result in serious harm or loss.

- Remain close to the bedside during the patient's emergence from general anesthesia because this can be a hazardous phase and you must continually monitor for potential or actual complications.

- Know in advance of need the location of the crash (code) cart and malignant hyperthermia supplies. This will save valuable time in the event of an emergency.

- Advise the anesthetist or OR nurse of any concerns or any questions you have about the patient before accepting responsibility for the patient. You should not assume care of the patient until you have the necessary information upon which to plan care. Efficient and effective patient care may suffer otherwise.

- Remind patients having any type of sedation that they may not drive, operate machinery, return to work, make important decisions or sign legal papers for 24-hours after receiving sedation. A few drugs have active metabolites that can have a second-peak effect and cause a return to drowsiness.

- Recover any patient who received ketamine (Ketalar) in a quiet place, because this drug can cause hallucinations in the postop period. A quiet atmosphere of "skillful neglect" can smooth the postanesthesia course and reduce the incidence of side effects.

- Always assist the patient when he or she stands the first time after a procedure; more than one assistant may be required for large patients. Orthostatic hypotension is not uncommon and may cause the patient to fall. Falls may also result from the effects of sedatives or the surgery.

- Be careful when applying an oxygen face mask to the face of the GA patient, because damage to the eyes or corneas can result from the straps or the mask.

- Do not extubate any patient who was reported difficult to intubate, because maintaining the airway may be difficult in the case of respiratory distress. Notify the anesthetist when the patient is ready to extubate.

- Check for bladder distention by palpating the abdomen in the patient who had a spinal or epidural anesthetic, because the patient may not be aware of a distended bladder. Notify the anesthetist and/or surgeon if the patient is unable to void after these regional anesthetics.

- Monitor the affected body parts in the patient who had regional or local anesthesia, because the patient may not be aware of discomfort and patient injury can result. For example, the patient may not be able to tell you that the ice pack is too cold or his legs are misaligned.

- Keep the side rails up on the bed. This helps prevent a fall and potential injury.

- Separate recovering children from adults whenever possible, because children may cry during emergence and this can disrupt other patient's recoveries.

- Move retching and vomiting patients away from other recovering patients when possible because this can stimulate the same response in other patients and may distress some patients.

# SUMMARY

This chapter focused generally on the care of the ambulatory patient immediately after the procedure, and more specifically on the care of the postanesthesia patient. After reviewing the usual progression of recovery from the different types of anesthesia, this chapter described general nursing care of the patient immediately after the procedure and then listed specific nursing strategies you can employ when caring for the ambulatory patient. Common postoperative complaints of the ambulatory patient were also addressed.

# CRITICAL CONCEPTS

- Maintenance of the airway, breathing, and circulation are the first priority in the PACU.

- Do not leave an unconscious patient unattended.

- Patients standing for the first time after the procedure must have assistance.

- Recovery from anesthesia is not an abrupt but a gradual process and it varies from one patient to another.

- Nurses assume a tremendous amount of responsibility in caring for postanesthesia patients; nurses caring for these patients need knowledge, expertise, and skill in postanesthesia nursing.

# EXAM QUESTIONS

## Chapter 9

Questions 50-57

50. Upon arrival in the postanesthesia care unit (PACU), the nurse should first assess the patient's:

    a. circulation
    b. awareness
    c. muscle tone
    d. airway

51. In caring for a patient who received ketamine (Ketalar), the PACU nurse should use:

    a. constant vigilance
    b. skillful neglect
    c. total assistance
    d. continuous care

52. Which of the following non-pharmacologic methods may prove helpful in reducing the sensation of nausea during the postoperative period?

    a. position changes
    b. cold wet towels to the patient's face and neck
    c. warm soaks to the wound
    d. icepacks to the neck

53. Patients should not drive for 24 hours after receiving sedatives because some medications have what kind of effect?

    a. second-peak
    b. latent onset
    c. delayed action
    d. primary cause

54. When standing for the first time after surgery, patients often experience:

    a. malignant hyperthermia
    b. orthostatic hypotension
    c. cardiac arrhythmias
    d. benign hypertension

55. Which of the following might happen in the PACU if an oxygen face mask was carelessly slipped on the unconscious patient's face?

    a. aspiration pneumonia
    b. orthostatic hypotension
    c. censory deprivation
    d. corneal abrasions

56. The final phase of general anesthesia is:

    a. Iinduction
    b. maintenance
    c. emergence
    d. delirium

57. Common complications in the PACU include pain, nausea and vomiting, and:

    a. malignant hyperthermia
    b. benign hypertension
    c. hypothermia
    d. hypoxia

# CHAPTER 10

# DISCHARGING THE PATIENT

## CHAPTER OBJECTIVE

After completing this chapter, you should be better prepared to discharge the ambulatory patient.

## LEARNING OBJECTIVES

After reading this chapter, you should be able to:

1. Identify nursing actions that enhance the comfort and safety of the patient as he or she is prepared for discharge.

2. Select potential nursing diagnoses for the ambulatory patient preparing for discharge.

3. Identify criteria for discharging ambulatory patients from the facility.

4. Recognize common complications that may require further intervention before the patient can be discharged.

## INTRODUCTION

The discharge of the patient from the ambulatory facility may be straightforward, especially if the procedure was minor and no anesthesia was involved. In this case, the patient is usually released when the procedure is complete, and no further intervention is necessary. But patients undergoing more complex procedures and surgery require careful evaluation and planning before discharge. Facilities vary in their policies about discharge, and this is an area that is still changing and will most likely continue to evolve as more health care delivery moves into the ambulatory sector. This chapter reviews assessment of the patient's readiness for discharge, common complications that may influence discharge, and the actual discharge of the patient. Nursing strategies for discharging the ambulatory patient are presented. The chapter closes with a summary and a review of the critical concepts.

## RECOVERY PHASE 2

Preparation for discharge begins before the patient is admitted to the ambulatory facility, because as is always true in health care, that which is not easily treated needs to be prevented. A preadmission interview either in person or over the telephone allows the nurse to gather information essential to planning care; this preadmission interview serves to identify potential concerns that could later turn into complications. These complications may necessitate canceling the case, delaying discharge, or admitting the patient to the hospital. Incidents such as these interfere with the delivery of quality care, frustrate the professional staff, and at the very least inconvenience patients. Clearly, planning for discharge begins when the patient is scheduled for ambulatory care.

## Nursing assessment

The nursing process is ideally initiated before the patient arrives at the ambulatory facility for care. This is especially true for patients having surgery with general anesthesia (GA) or regional anesthesia (RA). During this assessment, potential problem areas are identified and the patient is instructed in anticipated perioperative events. Issues that should be resolved before the patient is admitted include who will be transporting the patient home after the procedure and who will be providing care in the home after surgery. The patient should also prepare the home for his or her return, including removing potentially dangerous objects that might cause a fall, and setting up an area for recuperation. This area should be convenient to a bathroom and easily accessible; negotiating stairs will be difficult for most postoperative patients.

It is presumed that by the time the patient reaches Phase 2 of recovery, these issues have been resolved. All that is left then is for the nurse to assess the patient's readiness for discharge, teach home care, document the process, and discharge the patient. Most ambulatory units have predetermined criteria for discharge; this is usually based on a scoring system. See Fig. 10-1, for a Discharge Criteria form useful in assessing the patient's readiness to leave the facility. Factors scored in many systems include: vital signs, level of consciousness, pain control, voiding, mobility, condition of surgical site, and nutrition. You can double-check your assessment of the patient by evaluating the major body systems such as neurologic, cardiovascular, respiratory, or renal and noting how close the patient is to his or her preoperative baseline.

## Common complications

There are several relatively minor complications that may delay or preclude discharge, including nausea and vomiting, poorly controlled pain, and hypotension or syncope. When these cannot be adequately managed, ambulatory alternatives may provide the solution. These alternatives include overnight stay programs, observation units, assisted care facilities, or in some cases, hospitalization.

- Nausea and vomiting: N & V is still relatively common after anesthesia and surgery, but the incidence is decreasing with the introduction of new anesthetic agents. Both are generally well controlled by the use of antiemetics. Note that the sensation of nausea often accompanies hypotension and usually resolves when the blood pressure is raised. This is accomplished by infusion of a bolus of intravenous (IV) fluid or repositioning the patient; antiemetics are not usually necessary in this case. Sometimes N & V does not respond to treatment. In this case, the patient, support person and physician will confer and decide if the patient should attempt to go home with some antiemetic medication (such as suppositories) or be admitted to the hospital. Some facilities require a patient to tolerate liquids by mouth before discharge, but this varies.

- Pain: Occasionally the surgical procedure was prolonged or more extensive than planned and the patient will not be able to achieve adequate pain control with oral analgesics. In this case, hospital admission may be necessary.

- Hypotension and syncope: It is not uncommon for patients to feel weak upon rising the first time after surgery or other ambulatory procedures. Gradually taking the patient from supine to semi-sitting to sitting to standing usually reduces the potential for syncope; this process must be gradual and the patient must have assistance. Insufficient fluid replacement during the perioperative period contributes to this; adequate fluid replacement to prevent orthostatic hypotension is usually well tolerated by healthy patients.

# CHAPTER 10 — DISCHARGING THE PATIENT

## ASSESSMENT OF DISCHARGE CRITERIA (ADULT)

| Discharge Criteria and Score | | TIME | | | | | | |
|---|---|---|---|---|---|---|---|---|
| Respirations | 2 Regular rhythm; rate between 12 and 28<br>1 Shallow/on oxygen; rate <12 or >28<br>0 Dyspnea; rate <10 or >40 | | | | | | | |
| Circulation | 2 Postop systolic BP ± 20mm preop BP<br>1 Postop systolic BP ± 20-50mm preop BP<br>0 Postop systolic BP ± 50mm preop BP | | | | | | | |
| Activity/Exercise | 2 Able to ambulate on own<br>1 Ambulate with assistance<br>0 Unable to ambulate | | | | | | | |
| Cognitive/Perceptual | 2 States discharge instructions<br>1 Answers simple questions<br>0 Sleepy | | | | | | | |
| | 2 Free of discomfort<br>1 Medicated for discomfort (PO)<br>0 Medicated for discomfort (IM) | | | | | | | |
| Nutritional | 2 Taking PO fluids without nausea, emesis<br>1 Taking sips of PO fluid/ice chips<br>0 Unable to take to fluids | | | | | | | |
| Elimination | 2 Void quantity sufficient in bathroom<br>1 Void quantity sufficient bedpan/urinal<br>0 Unable to void | | | | | | | |
| Bleeding | 2 No bleeding<br>1 Moderate amount of bleeding<br>0 Large amount of bleeding | | | | | | | |
| Minimum discharge score needed: 14 | | TOTALS | | | | | | |

Name of physician notified of score of 13 or less before discharge: _____
Name of responsible adult accompanying patient home: _____
Discharge Instructions: Written ⊓ Verbal ⊓ Given to: ⊓ Pt. ⊓ Escort
Date: _____ Discharge Time: _____ RN Signature: _____

## ASSESSMENT OF DISCHARGE CRITERIA (PEDIATRIC)

| Discharge Criteria and Score | | TIME | | | | | | |
|---|---|---|---|---|---|---|---|---|
| Respirations | 2 Appropriate rate and depth for age (birth to 3 mos: 30-40/min, 3 mos to age 4: 20-30/min, >age 4: 14-20/min)<br>0 Croupy, wheezing, retractions or cyanosis; any evidence of airway obstruction | | | | | | | |
| Circulation | 2 Rate appropriate for age with normal peripheral perfusion (birth to 6 mos: 120 to 150/min, 6 mos to age 4: 90-120/min, age 4: 70-100/min)<br>0 Sustained tachycardia, vasoconstriction or poor capillary refill | | | | | | | |
| Activity/Exercise | 2 Normal age-appropriate preop activity<br>1 Awake<br>0 Arouses with difficulty | | | | | | | |
| Cognitive/Perceptual | 2 Discomfort appropriate to procedure<br>1 Medicated for discomfort (PO)<br>0 Requires parenteral analgesic | | | | | | | |
| Nutritional | 2 Taking PO fluids without nausea, emesis<br>1 Taking sips of PO fluid/ice chips<br>0 Unable to take fluids | | | | | | | |
| Elimination | 2 Void quantity sufficient<br>0 Unable to void | | | | | | | |
| Bleeding | 2 No bleeding<br>0 Large amount of bleeding | | | | | | | |
| Minimum discharge score needed: 11 | | TOTALS | | | | | | |

Name of physician notified of score of 10 or less before discharge: _____
Name of responsible adult accompanying patient home: _____
Discharge Instructions: Written ⊓ Verbal ⊓ Given to: ⊓ Pt. ⊓ Escort
Date: _____ Discharge Time: _____ RN Signature: _____

**Figure 10-1.** Discharge Criteria Form.
*Source:* East Memphis Surgery Center, Memphis, TN

# DISCHARGE

When the patient meets criteria, the nurse discharges the patient. In some units, a physician evaluates the patient before discharge, and a few physicians personally evaluate the patient themselves before discharge. But in many cases, the nurse makes the decision and releases the patient. You reach this decision based on whether or not the patient meets the criteria and the results of your nursing assessment.

Because some patients and families are skeptical of ambulatory surgery and doubt that anybody could have surgery and safely return home that same day, the nurse's attitude must be positive and upbeat. Experienced ambulatory care nurses exude confidence that the patient will do well; this in turn boosts the confidence of the patient and support person. Likewise, hesitation and ambivalence on the nurse's part can breed distress and concern in the patient. So it's important that the nurse have confidence in his or her skills in ambulatory care, and that the patient and support person believe discharge is the first step on the journey back to the patient's previous level of wellness.

Before leaving the facility, the patient and support person should have and understand instructions: transportation, when to call the doctor, when to return for follow-up care (if any), how to take medications, diet, activity restrictions, care of orthopedic devices if indicated, and wound or dressing care.

**Transportation.** Patients who received sedation or general anesthesia are never allowed to drive themselves home. This is because their judgment could be impaired and they could injure someone, including themselves. Most facilities will also not allow the patient to leave alone in a taxicab, because a responsible adult should accompany him or her to insure safe arrival in the home.

**Support person.** Patients undergoing surgery and general or regional anesthesia should have a responsible adult stay with them for at least 24 hours after surgery. This is not only a comfort measure, but a safety measure as well if complications arise. When patients claim no family or friend is available to assist them, home health agencies can be contacted to provide a paid caregiver. This support person should be able to meet the expected needs of the patient, such as assisting the patient to the bathroom if necessary. If the support person is, in the nurse's opinion, unsuitable as the caregiver, the nurse should explain this to the patient and notify the physician if a suitable substitute cannot be found.

**Physician follow-up.** Patients should have their doctor's number and be instructed in how to contact him or her in the event of a complication. They should also know when to return to the physician's office for follow-up care. Common indications for notifying the doctor after discharge include unrelieved pain or vomiting, inability to urinate, and excessive or unexpected bleeding. In the patient with a cast or bandage on an extremity, the patient should know to call the doctor if there is swelling, discoloration, or altered sensation in the extremity.

**Medications.** The patient should have a list of all medications along with how and when the drug(s) should be taken. Some states require patients to receive instructions on what the medication is, how it works, why it is prescribed, and the possible side effects.

**Diet.** The doctor generally specifies any special diet the patient must follow. In ambulatory surgery, the diet the patient consumed preoperatively is usually gradually resumed postoperatively. Patients who had sedation or general anesthesia should advance cautiously back to a regular diet; this means starting with water, then moving on to other liquids such as a soft drink or broth, then to well tolerated solids such as crackers, before returning to a full diet. Warn the patient about the dangers of consuming alcohol postoperatively; alcohol's negative effects are even more dangerous when combined with other drugs, including narcotics and transquilizers the patient may be taking postop.

**Activity.** The physician should specify any restrictions on the patient's activities and mobility. Otherwise, patients are generally allowed to return to activities gradually as tolerated. An exception is patients who have had general anesthesia or sedation. These patients should not drive, operate machinery, sign legal documents, or make important decisions for 24 hours after anesthesia or sedation.

**Wound care.** Specific instructions should be given to the surgical patient about dressings and care of the wound if indicated. These instructions will vary widely depending on the physician and the type of surgery.

**Other.** Instruct patients, where indicated, in care of casts, slings, or in activities such as crutch walking. Tell the patient the importance of follow-up care in the physician's office if indicated. Use this opportunity to educate the patient in good health habits and in the importance of following-up on any problems detected such as hypertension.

## Table 10-1
## Potential Nursing Diagnoses for the Patient Preparing for Discharge

| *Nursing Diagnosis* | *Sample nursing interventions* |
| --- | --- |
| Self-care deficits: hygiene, dressing, feeding, related to postop status | Advise patient preoperatively to wear loose fitting clothing and comfortable shoes that can be easily donned for the trip home and easily removed. Assist with dressing to go home. Instruct support person in patient's anticipated needs, such as assistance with getting to bathroom. Allow patient and support person time to ask questions and express concerns that you can then address. Do not release the postoperative patient to an adult who is unable to provide care. |
| Pain, related to ambulatory procedure | Administer analgesics as ordered, instruct patient and support person in administration of oral analgesics. Advise patient to avoid aspirin or aspirin-like drugs such as ibuprofen after surgery (because these products may cause bleeding) unless ordered by doctor. Tell patient the pain is expected to lessen, not worsen. Use non-pharmologic methods such as application of heat or ice, position changes, and massage if consistent with physician's orders. |
| Knowledge deficit, related to lack of exposure | Teach patient and support person about care required at home; validate their understanding and provide reinforcement in the form of written instructions. Give clear concise explanations, using terminology appropriate to level of understanding. Maintain a positive attitude about the patient and support person's ability to manage aftercare; stress benefits of ambulatory care, such as returning home to familiar environment. |

Please note this is a sample of potential nursing diagnoses and is not presented as, nor intended to be, a complete care plan for the ambulatory patient. More complete information can be found in a medical surgical nursing course and textbook.

Adapted from: *Nursing Diagnosis Reference Manual* by Sheila Sparks and Cynthia M. Taylor, Springhouse Corporation, 1991, and *Overview of Anesthesia* for Nurses by L. Chitwood, Western Schools, 1992.

In the event that the patient, for whatever reason, is unable to go home and must be transferred to a hospital, you should be supportive of the patient and family, offer explanations as necessary, prepare the patient for transfer, and give a complete report to the receiving nurse. Unplanned admissions usually dismay the patient and concern the family or support person, so support and empathy are essential during this time.

## FOLLOW-UP CARE

Many ambulatory facilities telephone the patient a day or two after surgery to evaluate the patient's progress and get feedback from the patient on the care provided. This is especially important in ambulatory surgery for the obvious reason that the patient is at home and not in the hospital where the nurse can perform a bedside assessment. During this interview, which is ideally conducted by the nurse, complications can be identified and the patient advised in further action if necessary. You are likely to find more consistent follow-up evaluations in the future, because health care facilities will find such evaluations to be an essential part of quality control and documentation of their care. Fig. 10-2 is a good example of a follow-up record.

## NURSING STRATEGIES

Discharging the ambulatory patient from an ambulatory unit is complex; detailed information can be found in medical and surgical textbooks. Below however, are basic nursing strategies and the rationale behind each. These should prove helpful as you care for a patient after an ambulatory procedure. As always, your intervention should be within the scope of your institution's practice guidelines, consistent your state's Nurse Practice Act and your license, and commensurate with your skills and training.

- Note that competent adult ambulatory patients who receive no anesthesia or sedation, or only local anesthesia, in most cases do not require an adult to accompany them home.

- Provide assistance to the patient as he or she attempts to stand for the first time. The number of personnel assisting should be proportionate to the patient's size and anticipated impairment. Many patients will feel weak and may suffer orthostatic hypotension and subsequent syncope upon standing the first time after surgery; having adequate assistance available may prevent a patient fall and injury.

- Involve the patient's support person in the care of the patient as soon as possible. This gives the support person some time to begin to feel comfortable with the patient's condition, to ask questions as necessary, and to begin to practice any skills that will be required as he or she provides continued home care for the patient.

- Insure privacy and confidentiality for the patient as he or she dresses for discharge and as you give discharge instructions. These are fundamental patient rights.

- Ascertain that the patient and support person have and understand written instructions about home care. The patient and the support person must understand aftercare before they are released because this is essential to continued care and avoidance of complications. Written instructions reinforce verbal instructions and provide valuable information such as names of medications and the physician's telephone number in the event of emergency.

- Gradually change the patient's position from supine to reclining to sitting to standing as you

# CHAPTER 10 —
## DISCHARGING THE PATIENT

113

|  | IMPRINT THIS AREA |
|---|---|
| SAINT FRANCIS HOSPITAL<br>5959 PARK AVENUE<br>MEMPHIS, TENNESSEE, 38119-5198<br>TELEPHONE: (901) 765-1000<br>**G I LABORATORY** | |

**Patient Name** _____  **Date:** _____

You have had an outpatient procedure. This procedure often involves intravenous sedation. Certain precautions need to be taken and instructions followed regarding your procedure. Indicated below by a check mark are instructions which need to be followed:

1. **Activity**
   _____ May resume normal activity _____.
   _____ Rest today, normal activity tomorrow as tolerated.
   _____ No heavy lifting for the next _____ day(s).
   _____ In reference to your endoscopic procedure, you may return to work.
   _____ Do not drive a vehicle, operate hazardous equipment or appliances for at least 24 hours after your procedure.
   _____ Refrain from making any complex decisions or executing any legal documents for at least 24 hours after your procedure.
   _____ Do not drink alcohol for at least 24 hours after your procedure.

2. **Diet**
   _____ Resume prior diet.
   _____ Low residue diet.
   _____ Decaffeinate prior diet.
   _____ Other _____.

3. **Medications**
   _____ May take all previous medications.
   _____ EXCEPTIONS: Advised against salicylates; aspirin containing compounds; and avoidance of arthritis medication.
   _____ Prescription(s) attached.
   _____ Other _____.

4. **Follow-up Appointment With Physician**
   _____ See physician on _____. Call office for appointment for further GI consultation.
   _____ See primary care physician, Dr. _____ in _____ days, _____ weeks.

5. **Special Instructions**
   _____ Observe for excessive bleeding or abnormal bleeding.
   _____ Persistent chills or fever over 101 degrees orally (use thermometer, don't guess).
   _____ If you were given medication in your vein it is not unusual to get redness and tenderness at the site of entry. If this does occur, place a warm washcloth at the site 2 to 3 times a day for a period of 20 minutes. The redness and tenderness will go away.

**IF THE ABOVE STATED SYMPTOMS ARE EXPERIENCED PLEASE CALL THE OFFICE.**

My post procedure instructions have been explained to me. I understand their content and a copy has been given to me. I have a responsible adult to drive me home.

_____   _____
Patient and/or responsible party                         Relationship

_____   _____  _____
Nurse                                                     Date           Time

**Figure 10–2.** Follow-Up Record.
*Source:* Saint Francis Hospital, Memphis, TN.

- prepare him or her for discharge; this will allow the circulatory system time to adapt and reduces the chance of orthostatic hypotension and syncope.

- Remind patients that even though they might feel recovered from the effects of sedation or anesthesia, they must still refrain from driving, operating machinery, signing legal documents, returning to work, or making important decisions for 24 hours. This is because some of these medications have active metabolites that may cause an unexpected return to drowsiness. Tell parents of children who have had anesthesia that the child should not ride a bike, play on gyms, ride skateboards, or engage in other activities or sports requiring coordination during this time, because injury could result.

- Explain to the patient that total absence of pain after a surgical procedure is neither an especially desirable nor a realistic goal. Patients should know that pain is an essential protective mechanism and it can seldom be completely eradicated.

- Note that the patient who complains of nausea after standing or being raised to a sitting position often is experiencing hypotension. The nausea results from decreased perfusion of the brain and is usually relieved by raising the blood pressureeither by returning the patient to a supine or trendelenburg position, or by an intravenous fluid bolus.

- Tell patients that if they are in doubt about whether a postoperative symptom warrants a call to their doctor, they should err on the side of caution and phone the physician. This may help catch a complication before it is serious.

- Remind patients to avoid alcoholic drinks for at least 24 hours after surgery, because alcohol is a drug that may interact with analgesics and other drugs to produce undesirable side effects, including coma or death.

- Tell patients that if they experience symptoms they believe indicate a true emergency, such as difficulty breathing or excessive bleeding from the wound, they should go immediately to the nearest emergency room for evaluation; their doctor can be notified from there. Patients should know this so they will not delay seeking treatment for potentially life threatening conditions.

- Instruct patients and their support person to notify the doctor if a swollen bruise appears over the incision. This is often a postoperative hematoma that will require intervention.

- Reassure the patient and support person that the patient will not be discharged until he or she has met all criteria and in the judgment of the staff is ready for discharge. Tell them that other patients undergoing similar procedures have done well after discharge. This can help boost their confidence.

- Do not release the postoperative surgery patient to the care of an adult who is unable or unwilling, for whatever reason, to provide responsible care. The patient may suffer harm in this case and alternative arrangements should be made.

- Do not release a child into the custody of an adult who is in your opinion unable or unwilling to provide the care the child needs to weather the postoperative course. Doing so could place the child at risk. Insure that the person who leaves with the child is indeed the legal guardian or custodial parent.

- Advise the nursing supervisor if the patient indicates dissatisfaction or anger about the care provided. The supervisor may choose to notify the physician, and in some cases should notify the institution's risk management department. Anger and dissatisfaction usually indicate that the patient's expectations were not met; learning the source of the complaint can help the facility meet or address those needs. Dissatisfied patients may turn to the courts to gain redress.

- Stress the positive benefits of ambulatory care: less time away from family and familiar environment, more relaxed and comfortable atmosphere for recovery. Patients and their support persons often adopt the nurse's attitude and will feel more confident if the nurse demonstrates confidence.

- Remind the postoperative patient that the pain lessens; the immediate postoperative pain is generally the most intense the pain will get. This can help reassure the patient that he or she should achieve adequate pain relief from oral analgesics and helps reduce "what if" anxiety centered around pain.

- Do not apply the fentanyl transdermal system (Duragesic) to ambulatory patients. It is contraindicated in the management of acute or postoperative pain, including ambulatory surgery; life threatening hypoventilation might occur. Duragesic has been implicated in ambulatory patient deaths, including a 9-year-old after tonsillectomy and a 17-year-old after widom teeth extraction (Janssen Pharmaceutica, 1-17 1994 letter). Duragesic is intended for the management or severe chronic pain, such as that associated with malignancy.

- Maintain intravenous access until recovery from anesthesia is complete, because complications could still arise, or intravenous fluid may be necessary to combat dehydration if vomiting develops.

- Obtain the signature of the patient or their support person acknowledging that they have received your instructions. This is documentation of your care for the patient's record.

# SUMMARY

Patients are undergoing more complex procedures and surgery; they require careful evaluation and planning before discharge. This chapter reviewed assessment of the patient's readiness for discharge, common complications that may influence discharge, and the actual discharge of the patient. Nursing strategies for use when discharging the ambulatory patient were presented.

# CRITICAL CONCEPTS

- Follow your facility's policy and guidelines when discharging ambulatory patients.

- Maintain a positive attitude about the patient and support person's ability to manage at home.

- Do not allow a patient who had sedation or anesthesia to drive home.

- Provide written instructions that reinforce your teaching to the patient and support person.

- Nurses assume a significant amount of responsibility in discharging patients from ambulatory care.

# EXAM QUESTIONS

# Chapter 10

Questions 58-63

58. After ambulatory surgery, children are released into the care of their:

   a. guardian or custodial parent
   b. probation officer
   c. teacher or neighbor
   d. friend

59. Patients not allowed to drive themselves home after an ambulatory procedure include those who had:

   a. no sedation
   b. general anesthesia
   c. local anesthesia
   d. no medications

60. A new analgesic that is contraindicated in ambulatory surgery is:

   a. nalbuphine (Nubain)
   b. meperidine (Demerol)
   c. morphine sulfate
   d. fentanyl transdermal system (Duragesic)

61. As you assess your hernia patient before discharge, you note a swollen bruise is developing at the incision. You notify the surgeon because this is most likely a:

   a. postoperative hematoma
   b. collapsed lung
   c. postoperative abscess
   d. latent infection

62. As you conduct discharge teaching for your patient who had an arthroscopy, you explain that he must not ingest alcoholic drinks while he is taking narcotic analgesics because which of the following may develop?

   a. hypothermia
   b. tuberculosis
   c. priapism
   d. coma

63. Patients who experience symptoms (such as excessive bleeding or difficulty breathing) after discharge that they believe indicate a true emergency should first:

   a. call their doctor
   b. go to the nearest hospital emergency room
   c. return to the ambulatory facility
   d. notify the nurse

# CHAPTER 11

# SPECIAL AMBULATORY PATIENTS

## CHAPTER OBJECTIVE

After completing this chapter, you should be better prepared to differentiate among and deliver care to ambulatory patients who have special needs.

## LEARNING OBJECTIVES

After reading this chapter, you should be able to:

1. Identify patients who may require special attention from the ambulatory team.

2. Choose methods of modifying nursing care to meet the special needs of these patients.

3. Recognize common analgesics prescribed for pediatric patients.

4. Recognize complications that may develop in the ambulatory geriatric and pediatric patient.

5. Select nursing strategies that may be effective for ambulatory trauma (non-life threatening) patients and emergency surgery patients.

## INTRODUCTION

This chapter provides an overview of the care of patients who may have special nursing needs: children, the impaired, the elderly, and trauma or emergency patients. Every patient is entitled to the best possible care no matter what his habitus, so when this chapter refers to these patients' special nursing needs, you should not infer that they should somehow get better care than other patients. It does mean that in nursing these patients, you may find unique, individual, or extraordinary needs or circumstances that require modifications in the nursing care plan. Many of these special patients have common needs, such as thermoregulation; many will have unique needs that you will identify and meet just for them. In the past, these patients might have been hospitalized so that their perioperative needs could be met by professionals. Now however, many of these patients are channeled into the ambulatory care system among the healthy patients. The nurse must be prepared to meet the challenge of providing care to these patients in ambulatory settings. Common concerns when caring for these special patients are briefly discussed in this chapter. More complete information and discussions can be found in pediatric, geriatric, and other specialty nursing textbooks. Nursing strategies are listed. A summary and a review of the critical concepts presented close the chapter.

# AMBULATORY PEDIATRIC PATIENTS

Ambulatory care is ideal for pediatric patients because it allows minimal disruption of the child's life and reduces anxiety caused by prolonged separations from the family. In fact, so many pediatric procedures can be completed on an ambulatory basis that there are diagnostic and surgical facilities designed specifically for children and staffed by professionals specializing in pediatrics. It is not uncommon however, for children to come to facilities designed for adults, and the nurse must be prepared to meet the needs of these pediatric patients. Remember that children are not simply miniature versions of adults; you should know normal ranges and values for vital signs and other parameters in children because this is essential for nursing care. For example, a heart rate of 70 in a newborn is cause for alarm, but is normal in an adult. Preparation for caring for pediatric patients should include review of a pediatric nursing textbook; the discussion presented here is simply an overview of common basic concerns. It is also prudent to note that just because they are small, children are no less important; children should receive the same high standard of care that you would give an adult.

## Preparation

Pediatric patients seem to benefit from a preoperative visit to the ambulatory center a few days before their procedure. These children may take a brief tour of the facility, and may even practice breathing from the "magic space mask" (anesthesia mask) while there. Meeting the staff also serves to reduce the child's anxiety.

Before beginning any pediatric procedure, make certain all equipment and supplies are available. Any ambulatory facility performing pediatric procedures must have pediatric equipment. While this might seem obvious, you should determine that emergency equipment and supplies are in the facility before starting any procedure.

When caring for the pediatric patient, you must also integrate the parents into the care plan. Children often take their cues from their parents, so an anxious parent can result in an anxious child. Enlist the parent's help in caring for the child and tell them what to expect.

- Preoperative fasting: The length of time the pediatric patient must be NPO before anesthesia varies; follow your institution's or anesthetist's policy. Caution parents to strictly enforce the NPO policy because cancellation or aspiration could result from non-compliance.

- Preoperative sedation: Pediatric anesthetists and pediatricians vary widely in their opinion and usage of preoperative sedation. Many children coming for brief procedures such as tubes in the ears receive no preoperative medication. This enables the child to return promptly to the parents in most cases. However, preoperative medication may be ordered by the anesthetist or surgeon. Some order injections of sedatives or anticholinergic drugs; some order syrups containing tranquilizers such as midazolam (Versed); some have the nurse administer midazolam or the narcotic sufentanil (Sufenta) into the child's nose; some offer the narcotic fentanyl (Sublimaze) in a lollipop; some use rectal instillation of a barbiturate or other drug with a sedating action. Ketamine (Ketalar), a phencyclidine discussed in Chapter 5, is more commonly used in pediatrics than in adult care. Ketamine sedates the patient and produces analgesia, but can have unpleasant side effects such as nightmares and hallucinations. Some facilities are using a new preparation, eutetic mixture of local anesthetics (EMLA) to facilitate IV insertion in the conscious child. This cream is applied at the site about 60 minutes before IV insertion; it anesthetizes the skin.

- Preoperative play: Allowing children to play with an anesthesia mask or a surgical cap or mask gives them an opportunity to act out some of their concerns. There are coloring and story books available about going to the doctor or hospital that may help some children cope with anxiety.

- Separation: A few facilities will allow a parent to be present during part or all of an ambulatory procedure, or during the induction of anesthesia. In other situations, the child is separated from the parents as diplomatically as is possible, although inevitably some separations are turbulent.

## During the procedure

When small children are anesthetized for surgery, they frequently sit in the anesthetist's lap or on the operating room (OR) table for an inhalation induction. A pulse oximeter is attached to a finger or toe if the child will allow it. An anesthesia mask, pleasantly flavored with a fruit (strawberry, cherry, etc.) or bubble gum scent, is held near the child's face so the child begins to inhale the anesthetic agent. As induction continues, the mask is sealed against the child's face, and the patient is laid down on the OR table. Monitoring is started. Intravenous (IV) access is secured in all but brief procedures, and then the physician begins work. Sometimes the induction is not so smooth or playful; the team must use their professional judgment when deciding to forcibly restrain a child for induction or abort the induction. Establishing anesthesia via this inhalation induction (as opposed to an IV induction) means the patient will travel through several planes of anesthesia before reaching surgical anesthesia. The child will pass through an excitement phase, which often includes some struggling and breath holding, although the patient should not remember any of this.

Older (9-10 years of age) children or mature children may cooperate with establishing an IV before the procedure. In this case, an IV induction can be performed, thereby avoiding the perils of an inhalation induction, and progressing directly to surgical anesthesia.

- Thermoregulation: Children, especially infants, have limited thermoregulatory capacity and will become hypothermic quickly in a cold procedure room. The room should be warmed before the patient enters; warming devices will have to be used unless the procedure is brief. Hypothermia can slow recovery.

- Fluid balance: When admitting a pediatric patient, obtain an accurate weight and height and document this on the chart. Convert pounds to kilograms (kg) with the method presented in Chapter 7 or divide pounds by 2.2 to determine kg; basic drug dosages and fluid administration are calculated based on weight in kg. Inadvertent administration of excessive IV fluids can result in a child's death, so IV infusions must be monitored carefully.

- Monitoring: Children should receive the same monitoring that an adult would, and temperature must be closely monitored to prevent the development of hypothermia.

## Aftercare

Many pediatric facilities reunite parents with their children as soon as possible after a procedure, because a familiar person is generally better able to soothe any distress.

- Pain management: It is unconscionable to deny infants and children analgesics during and after painful procedures; the inability to verbalize pain does not mean that it doesn't exist or isn't severe. Some children will not report pain to a nurse for fear of a "shot," so you will have to work with the parent to determine when the child is hurting and the best method to relieve it. Table 11-1, Dosing Data, lists dosages for common analgesics. This is provided only as a reference for you; always check current prescribing information and be aware that the patient's condition may require adjustment in doses. Fig. 11-1 lists critical questions to consider before and during pharmacologic management of pain in children.

- Home instructions: Parents will need careful instruction in home care; this information should be given to them in written form. Because parents may be anxious about their ability to provide necessary home care, determine that they do indeed comprehend instructions before releasing them from the facility, then reassure them.

# AMBULATORY GERIATRIC PATIENTS

In 1900, the elderly (people over 65) constituted 4% of the population. By 1988, that proportion was up to 12.4 %, by 2000 it will be 13% and by 2030, 22%. The most rapid population increase over the next decade will be among those over 85 years of age (Healthy People 2000). These patients are currently covered by Medicare, a government entitlement health care program; many of these patients will be treated as ambulatory. The nurse can expect then, to see increasing numbers of elderly in ambulatory facilities.

Aging is a normal, not pathologic process. In general, aging results in a decline in the body's reserve functioning, so there is less margin of error. For ex-

---

- Have the child and parent(s) been asked about their previous experiences with pain and their preferences for use of analgesics?
- Is the child being adequately assessed at appropriate intervals?
- Are analgesics ordered for prevention and relief of pain?
- Is the analgesic strong enough for the pain expected or the pain being experienced?
- Is the timing of drug administration appropriate (preferably oral or intravenous) for the child?
- Is the child adequately monitored for the occurrence of side effects?
- Are side effects appropriately managed?
- Has the analgesic regimen provided adequate comfort and satisfaction from the child's or parents' perspective?

Parallel questions regarding nonpharmacologic strategies include:
- Have the child and parent(s) been asked about their experiences with and preferences for a given strategy?
- Is the strategy appropriate for the child's developmental level, condition, and type of pain?
- Is the timing of the strategy sufficient to optimize its effects?
- Is the strategy adequately effective in preventing or alleviating the child's pain?
- Are the child and parent(s) satisfied with the strategy for prevention or relief of pain?
- Are the treatable sources of emotional distress for the child being addressed?

**Figure 11-1.** Critical Questions Regarding the Adequacy of Pain Management Strategies

*Source*: Acute Pain Management Guideline Panel. *Acute Pain Management: Operative or Medical Procedures and Trauma.* Clinical Practice Guideline. AHCPR Pub. No. 92-0032. Rockville, MD: Agency for Health Care Policy and Research, Public Health Service, U. S. Department of Health and Human Services. Feb. 1992.

# Table 11-1
## Dosing Data for Opioid Analgesics

| Drug | Approximate equianalgesic oral dose | Approximate equianalgesic parenteral dose | Recommended starting dose (adults more than 50 kg body weight) oral | Recommended starting dose (adults more than 50 kg body weight) parenteral | Recommended starting dose (children and adults less than 50 kg body weight)[1] oral | Recommended starting dose (children and adults less than 50 kg body weight)[1] parenteral |
|---|---|---|---|---|---|---|
| **Opioid Agonist** | | | | | | |
| Morphine[2] | 30 mg q 3–4 hr (around-the-clock dosing) 60 mg q 3–4 hr (single dose or intermittent dosing) | 10 mg q 3–4 hr | 30 mg q 3–4 hr | 10 mg q 3–4 hr | 0.3 mg/kg q 3–4 hr | 0.1 mg/kg q 3–4 hr |
| Codeine[3] | 130 mg q 3–4 hr | 75 mg q 3–4 hr | 60 mg q 3–4 hr | 60 mg q 2 hr (intramuscular/subcutaneous) | 1 mg/kg q 3–4 hr[4] | Not recommended |
| Hydromophone[2] (Dilaudid) | 7.5 mg q 3–4 hr | 1.5 mg q 3–4 hr | 6 mg q 3–4 hr | 1.5 mg q 3–4 hr | 0.06 mg/kg q 3–4 hr | 0.015 mg/kg q 3–4 hr |
| Hydrocodone (in Lorcet, Lortab, Vicodin, others) | 30 mg q 3–4 hr | Not available | 10 mg q 3–4 hr | Not available | 0.2 mg/kg q 3–4 hr[4] | Not available |
| Levorphanol (Levo-Dromoran) | 4 mg q 6–8 hr | 2 mg q 6–8 hr | 4 mg q 6–8 hr | 2 mg q 6–8 hr | 0.04 mg/kg q 6–8 hr | 0.02 mg/kg q 6–8 hr |
| Meperidine (Demerol) | 300 mg q 2–3 hr | 100 mg q 3 hr | Not recommended | 100 mg q 3 hr | Not recommended | 0.75 mg/kg q 2–3 hr |
| Methadone (Dolophine, others) | 20 mg q 6–8 hr | 10 mg q 6–8 hr | 20 mg q 6–8 hr | 10 mg q 6–8 hr | 0.2 mg/kg q 6–8 hr | 0.1 mg/kg q 6–8 hr |
| Oxycodone (Roxicodone, also in Percocet, Percodan, Tylox, others) | 30 mg q 3–4 hr | Not available | 10 mg q 3–4 hr | Not available | 0.2 mg/kg q 3–4 hr[4] | Not available |
| Oxymorphone[2] (Numorphan) | Not available | 1 mg q 3–4 hr | Not available | 1 mg q 3–4 hr | Not recommended | Not recommended |
| **Opioid Agonist-Antagonist and Partial Agonist** | | | | | | |
| Buprenorphine (Buprenex) | Not available | 0.3–0.4 mg q 6–8 hr | Not available | 0.4 mg q 6–8 hr | Not available | 0.004 mg/kg q 6–8 hr |
| Butorphanol (Stadol) | Not available | 2 mg q 3–4 hr | Not available | 2 mg q 3–4 hr | Not available | Not recommended |
| Nalbuphine (Nubain) | Not available | 10 mg q 3–4 hr | Not available | 10 mg q 3–4 hr | Not available | 0.1 mg/kg q 3–4 hr |
| Pentazocine (Talwin, others) | 150 mg q 3–4 hr | 60 mg q 3–4 hr | 50 mg q 4–6 hr | Not recommended | Not recommended | Not recommended |

**Note:** Published tables vary in the suggested doses that are equianalgesic to morphine. Clinical response is the criterion that must be applied for each patient; titration to clinical response is necessary. Because there is not complete cross tolerance among these drugs, it is usually necessary to use a lower than equianalgesic dose when changing drugs and to retitrate to response.

**Caution:** recommended doses do not apply to patients with renal or hepatic insufficiency or other conditions affecting drug metabolism and kinetics.

[1] **Caution:** Doses listed for patients with body weight less than 50 kg cannot be used as initial starting doses in babies less than 6 months of age. Consult the *Clinical Practice Guideline for Acute Pain Management: Operative or Medical Procedures and Trauma* section on management of pain in neonates for recommendations.

[2] For morphine, hydromorphone, and oxymorphone, rectal administration is an alternate route for patients unable to take oral medications, but equianalgesic doses may differ from oral and parenteral doses because of pharmacokinetic differences.

[3] **Caution:** Codeine doses above 65 mg often are not appropriate due to diminishing incremental analgesia with increasing doses but continually increasing constipation and other side effects.

[4] **Caution:** Doses of aspirin and acetaminophen in combination opioid/NSAID preparations must also be adjusted to the patient's body weight.

*Source:* Acute Pain Management Guideline Panel. *Acute Pain Management: Operative or Medical Procedures and Trauma.* Clinical Practice Guideline. AHCPR Pub. No. 92-0032. Rockville, MD: Agency for Health Care Policy and Research, Public Health Service, U. S. Department of Health and Human Services. Feb. 1992.

ample, the maximal breathing capacity is less, so hypoxia may develop quicker during a procedure. However, unlike children, the elderly are not as often in good health. Any disease processes must be taken into consideration and addressed whenever elderly patients come to the ambulatory unit.

## Preparation

The elderly usually need extra time during the ambulatory procedure because it often takes them a little longer to get where they're going, change clothes, and read or sign forms. The nurse may need to read forms to the elderly patient, or assist him or her in dressing.

- Preoperative sedation: Preoperative sedation is often not necessary; when used, it generally should be light for elderly patients and it should be tailored to each patient's condition.

- Medications: Many anesthetists now have the patient continue to take regularly scheduled medications with a sip ( cc) of water even while NPO for an upcoming procedure. This avoids disrupting vital medications that may be stabilizing the patient's condition.

## During the procedure

When caring for the elderly, you may find that you need to speak a little louder and a little slower to facilitate communication. You should also provide adequate warmth, because the elderly are subject to hypothermia, as are children. Because of their reduced metabolism, the elderly often require less sedation. Limited mobility and the presence of musculoskeletal disorders such as arthritis mean that the patient may require extra padding when positioned for an ambulatory procedure.

## Aftercare

Ambulatory care means the patient will return home that night, but this can be difficult for some ambulatory patients, especially those who live alone or with an elderly partner. As a nurse, you will have to determine whether this support person is capable of providing aftercare. In the event the support person appears incapable of providing home care, alternative arrangements must be made. This might including engaging a private duty home health attendant, admission to a hospital, or transfer to an extended care unit. The elderly should receive written instructions in print that is large enough for them to read, and you should make certain all aids removed from them for the procedure (hearing aids, dentures, canes, etc.) are returned before the patient is discharged.

# OTHER PATIENTS WITH SPECIAL NEEDS

With the trend towards ambulatory care, you can expect to see more patients with unique nursing needs. This might include impaired patients and victims of non-life threatening trauma or certain emergencies. While basic nursing diagnoses will be consistent with those for other ambulatory patients, you will often be able to identify other concerns. In general, when faced with patients requiring special care, try to allow extra time to care for them, and try to assign one nurse to the patient's care, without rotating different staff.

## Impaired patients

It is hoped that the nature of a patient's impairment will be made known in advance so special measures can be taken to meet the patient's needs by assigning additional staff and obtaining any special equipment that might be needed. As with other patients with chronic health concerns, regularly scheduled medications are often continued during the ambulatory period to maintain homeostasis.

- Physical impairment: Physical impairments may be relatively minor or extensive and may be associated with chronic disease. Some impairments may result in major modifications in anesthesia care, so the anesthesia team should be notified well in advance. Physically impaired patients may also require an attendant or other caregiver to be present constantly during the ambulatory period. In patients with congenital disorders, the nurse should note that where there is one defect, there may be more; an awareness of this potential helps in planning care. Patients with sensory impairments, such as blindness or deafness, can often guide you in how best to communicate with them. For example, the deaf person may request that you face him so he can read your lips.

- Mental impairment: Emotional or developmental impairment in a patient always results in special nursing needs. Empathy, patience, and a non-judgmental attitude are essential qualities of the nurse caring for these patients. The bedside presence of the patient's support person should be allowed as long as is possible during the ambulatory period.

## Trauma and emergency patients

Patients who have experienced non-life threatening trauma such as fractures or lacerations are often seen in minor emergency clinics which provide ambulatory care. Some of these patients will be subsequently referred to ambulatory surgical facilities for surgical correction. Other ambulatory units will admit patients from physicians' offices for emergency surgery for conditions such as appendicitis or ectopic pregnancy. The need for immediate intervention must be weighed against the risks of anesthesia in the trauma or emergency patient. Trauma and stress slow the emptying of the stomach, and many patients are so unnerved by what is happening that they frequently are unable to give a complete history of their medical condition or last ingestion of food or drink.

# NURSING STRATEGIES

The strategies for caring for an ambulatory patient with special needs are complex and numerous; detailed information can be found in medical and surgical nursing textbooks. Below however, are basic nursing strategies and the rationale behind each. As always, your intervention should be within the scope of your institution's practice guidelines, consistent your state's Nurse Practice Act and your license, and commensurate with your skills and training.

**Pediatrics:** The following are nursing strategies relevant to pediatric patients.

- Know in advance of need the location of the pediatric crash (code) cart and malignant hyperthermia supplies. This will save valuable time in the event of an emergency.

- Monitor IV infusions carefully in children, because sudden and unintended infusion of an excessive volume of IV fluid could result in the child's death. Many institutions use an electronic IV fluid controller to reduce the potential for this complication. Other methods include hanging the smallest possible container of IV fluid, such as 100-250 cc containers, or using an IV set with an in-line chamber that will only hold 50-100 cc at a time.

- Note that inhalation inductions in children, which usually begin by directing high flows of oxygen and nitrous oxide (along with the anesthetic agent) at the child's face before achieving a good seal with the mask, may significantly raise the levels of waste anesthetic gases in the OR. Some degree of contamination of the OR with the waste gases is unavoidable in pediatric inhalation inductions, but pregnant personnel should limit their exposure in these situations because of possible teratogenic effects. Intravenous inductions bypass this problem but not all children will tolerate IV insertion, and many professionals don't believe an IV is necessary for very brief procedures.

- Stress the positive aspects of the procedure to the child: getting out of school, getting to do something brothers or sisters do not, getting special attention, receiving hats, masks, and shoe covers to take home. Focusing on the positive may help the parent and child feel less fearful of the experience.

- Monitor closely the child who received preoperative sedation, because these are potent drugs that could cause respiratory depression, hypoxia and death.

- Don't threaten other children present with the patient. Telling children you will "give them a shot" if they misbehave infers that those receiving such health care interventions have been bad. Injections or other procedures are not disciplinary measures; implying otherwise will only make it more difficult the next time that child requires health care.

- Read and then re-read each physician's order for preoperative sedation for a child. Question any order that seems excessive or unusual; double-check your arithmetic when drawing up the medication; ask another nurse to check with you. These steps can help prevent error and tragedy. If you find yourself drawing up more than one vial or ampule of any drug, you're probably drawing up too much, check again.

- Take admission to the facility as an opportunity for teaching parents and older children about good health habits. Instruct parents in the value of preventive care; teach older children about the risks associated with abuse of substances such as food, nicotine, alcohol, and illicit drugs. Nurses have always been committed to health promotion and this is an excellent opportunity to guide young lives in good health habits.

- Tailor your assessment and nursing care to the child's developmental level and personality style. This can facilitate the delivery of that care.

- Accept the parent's report of pain when the child is unable or unwilling to report it himself. This helps avoid the development of severe pain and aids in your administration of analgesics.

- Provide maximum treatment for pain and anxiety during the first procedure for the child who is expected to have multiple procedures. This reduces anxiety during subsequent procedures.

- Prepare the child and parent for the procedure with developmentally appropriate materials. This will enhance understanding.

- Note that infants, especially those born prematurely, may be susceptible to apnea and may require respiratory or cardiac monitoring after a procedure to prevent a tragedy.

- Use non-pharmacologic methods to assist in pain relief for the pediatric surgical patient. Pacifiers, swaddling, rocking, holding, positioning, and the presence of familiar toys are common interventions. This may reduce the need for analgesics postoperatively.

- Know the ranges of normal vital signs for your pediatric patients. Normal blood pressures and heart rates differ for children and adults; knowledge of what is normal and what is not will help you identify areas for intervention.

**Geriatrics.** The following are nursing strategies relevant to geriatric patients:

- Ask geriatric patients to come to the ambulatory facility a little early since their preparation frequently takes a little longer.

- Be vigilant and provide assistance to the elderly patient when he or she ambulates. Falls are the second most common (auto accidents are first) cause of injury in the elderly and this potential can be high in a patient who has had sedation or is in unfamiliar surroundings.

- Allow geriatric patients to keep their sensory aids such as hearing aids or eyeglasses when possible. This enhances their comfort and facilitates your care.

- Note that many facilities allow elderly patients to keep their dentures in place if general anesthesia isn't planned. Dentures help maintain the airway by retaining its structure; patients are often more comfortable with their dentures in place.

- Place a warmed blanket on the stretcher before the patient is transferred to it and then cover the patient with another warmed blanket. This is a comfort as well as hypothermia reducing measure.

- Treat elderly patients as you do other patients: with respect. Avoid referring to the patient with unprofessional jargon such as "Gramps" or "Sweetie." While you may feel quite nurturing towards the patient, failure to address the patient in a professional manner is demeaning to the patient and can lead to dissatisfaction and anxiety.

- Take admission to the facility as an opportunity for teaching your patients about good health habits. Advise patients to seek treatment for concerns detected during admission such as high blood pressure or increased blood glucose. Explain the role of nutrition, exercise, and smoking cessation in good health.

**Impaired patients.** The following are nursing strategies relevant to impaired patients:

- Treat impaired patients with respect and maintain their dignity throughout the ambulatory period. Being treated with respect and dignity are fundamental patient rights. Impaired patients are no less valuable or important than patients who are not impaired, and they have the same rights, even when they are unable to speak for themselves.

- Act as the impaired patient's advocate to protect his or her rights. Patients with handicaps or deformities should be protected from curiosity seekers and others who have no role in their care.

- Use appropriate medical terminology when referring to a patient's impairment. Do not use slang terms like "cripple," "dumb," or "idiot." These labels are inaccurate and inappropriate; the family and patient are usually dismayed and angered to hear a professional using these terms.

- Give all patients the same high quality care, because that is your professional obligation as a nurse. Mentally impaired patients can still benefit from gentle touch and simple explanations, even when they are unable to respond as other patients might. Delivering the same high level of nursing care demonstrates respect for human life and helps remind other staff members that the patient is entitled to quality care and concern.

**Trauma and emergency patients.** The following are nursing strategies relevant to minor trauma and emergency patients seen in ambulatory units:

- Allow the patient time to express emotions about the incident that has brought him or her to the facility; this can reduce anxiety.

- Ask the patient to think carefully about any food intake before the accident, many patients will subsequently recall coffee or soft drinks they had before the emergency developed.

- Note that stress from an accident or sudden illness limits the patient and family's ability to comprehend information you give. Offer simple instructions and explanations and repeat often. This will help insure that the patient and family retain your teaching and it can reduce their anxiety.

- Reassure the patient and family that you are aware this is a difficult time for them and that you and the staff will do everything you can to reduce their distress and meet their needs. Such reassurances build their confidence in your care and may reduce their anxiety.

- Be aware that injuries to women and children may have been intentionally inflicted, often by someone known to the victim. Follow your facility's policy and your state's laws in reporting suspected family violence and assaults, and do not release a child or postoperative patient to a suspected abuser until an investigation has been completed. Doing so could result in further injury or death for the patient. This may mean admitting the patient to a hospital or extended care facility while an investigation is conducted.

# SUMMARY

This chapter provided an overview of the care of patients who may have special nursing needs: children, the impaired, the elderly, and trauma or emergency patients. It was noted that while all patients are entitled to quality professional care, these patients may have unique needs that require special intervention. Common concerns when caring for these special patients were briefly discussed in this chapter. Nursing strategies were listed.

# CRITICAL CONCEPTS

- All patients are entitled to respectful professional care regardless of their condition.

- Use caution when administering medication to children and the elderly because the margin of error is reduced. Ask another nurse to double-check orders and dosages with you.

- Pediatric and geriatric patients are especially susceptible to the negative effects of chilling and so must be protected from hypothermia.

- Infants and children feel pain and are entitled to relief from that pain.

# EXAM QUESTIONS

## Chapter 11

Questions 64-70

64. In which patient would a heart rate of 70 be a cause for alarm?

   a. 80-year old female
   b. *2-month old male*
   c. 7-year old male
   d. 19-year old female

65. A new product that can reduce the pain of IV insertion is:

   a. *eutetic mixture of local anesthetics (EMLA)*
   b. midazolam (Versed)
   c. regional propofol (Diprivan)
   d. desflurane (Suprane)

66. An anesthetic agent that is used mostly in children but that sometimes causes hallucinations and nightmares is:

   a. halothane (Fluothane)
   b. propofol (Diprivan)
   c. *ketamine (Ketalar)*
   d. midazolam (Versed)

67. In young children, anesthesia is usually induced by:

   a. *inhalation*
   b. intravenous injection
   c. rectal suppository
   d. nasal instillation

68. During the perioperative period, geriatric and pediatric patients are especially vulnerable to:

   a. hyperthermia
   b. hypotension
   c. *hypothermia*
   d. hypertension

69. While drawing up an injection for a child, you find that you have to open three ampules of the drug. You should:

   a. administer the injection
   b. *double-check the physician's orders and the medication label*
   c. disregard the order and discard the medication
   d. discuss the need for the injection with the parents

70. Inhalation inductions in children can:

   a. *contaminate the OR*
   b. cheer the OR staff
   c. relax the surgeon
   d. sterilize the OR

# CHAPTER 12

# AMBULATORY NURSING CONSIDERATIONS IN THE SURGICAL SPECIALTIES

## CHAPTER OBJECTIVE

After completing this chapter, you should be better prepared to implement the nursing process for ambulatory patients undergoing different types of surgery.

## LEARNING OBJECTIVES

After reading this chapter, you should be able to:

1. Select potential nursing diagnoses for each classification of patients within a surgical specialty.

2. Identify common needs of patients undergoing routine surgical procedures.

3. Choose methods to provide ambulatory nursing care to surgical patients based on the common nursing diagnoses and patient needs identified for that class of patients.

4. Specify nursing measures that enhance the probability of a favorable outcome after specialty surgery.

5. Recognize common complications that may develop based on the type of surgery.

## INTRODUCTION

Virtually all the surgical specialties perform at least some procedures in the ambulatory setting. While it is beyond the scope of this course to describe and review every ambulatory surgical procedure, the ambulatory patient care nurse should be familiar with the most common types of procedures performed in ambulatory surgical settings. This chapter briefly explores each of the surgical specialties and then groups common procedures into classifications. Grouping procedures into classifications can make it easier to understand the complications and concerns that are common to each group. This facilitates learning, expedites the planning and delivery of nursing care, and alerts you to search for more in-depth information as needed. This chapter closes with a summary and a list of the critical concepts presented.

# AMBULATORY SURGERY

As mentioned in Chapter 1, many surgical procedures are moving from inpatient to ambulatory settings; ophthalmology and gynecology are two surgical specialties especially well represented. For example, uncomplicated vaginal hysterectomies that just five years ago would have required 3-5 days hospitalization are now performed on an ambulatory basis, as are some cholecystectomies. Moving previously inpatient procedures into the ambulatory arena is aided by the development of facilities that specialize in just that care, such as plastic surgery or ophthalmology. When the staff is familiar with the procedure and supportive of the ambulatory philosophy, many operations are safely performed on an ambulatory basis. The key is that the staff be well trained and the patients carefully selected. Disaster may ensue when procedures are performed on patients in less than optimal condition by a staff not familiar with the procedure or with potential complications that might arise.

You probably already know that not all patients are enthusiastic about ambulatory surgery. The support person or family member who will be providing aftercare is often anxious and concerned about their ability to provide such care. In 1991 Caldwell found that common concerns of ambulatory surgical patients included uncertainty about possible malignancy (43.5%), fear of anesthesia (30.3%), and fear of pain or complications after discharge. Caldwell also found that some patients may perceive that the surgery is minor and the risks are lower if it is performed on an ambulatory basis.

So ambulatory surgical nurses face a number of challenges in implementing the nursing process for their patients. In the following sections, each of the surgical specialty fields will be explored and common procedures with associated nursing diagnoses will be grouped into classifications. Grouping procedures into classes can make it easier to understand complications and concerns that are common to each group. This should facilitate your learning and recall, because rather than attempting to memorize specific procedures and nursing actions, you are able to note the common nursing diagnoses and implement the nursing process from that point. Knowing the basics of each group of procedures also serves to alert you to search for more in-depth information as you need it.

# GYNECOLOGY AND OBSTETRICS

Launched into the ambulatory arena with the introduction of lasers and laparoscopes, many gynecologic and a few obstetric procedures are well suited to the ambulatory setting, since these technologic advances reduce the need for opening the abdomen to diagnose or treat. Gynecologic surgery is quite commonly performed in ambulatory units; a number of minor procedures are even done in the gynecologist's office. Occasionally a procedure that could be done in the gynecologist's office is performed in the ambulatory surgery unit under general anesthesia, due to patient intolerance. This may include simple procedures such as a pelvic exam or Pap smear; the patient is usually young and anxious. Pregnant patients are also seen in ambulatory units, most often for elective abortion or treatment of spontaneous abortion (miscarriage) and ectopic (tubal) pregnancy. Most gynecologic surgical procedures require either general (GA) or regional (epidural or spinal) anesthesia (RA). Common gynecologic procedures are grouped into several classifications below: intra-abdominal, intrauterine, cervical or vaginal, and genital. Your patient may be having one or more of these procedures at the same time.

## Intra-abdominal surgery

In the past, intra-abdominal surgery meant an incision, manipulation of the pelvic organs, significant postoperative pain, a hospital stay, and weeks of recovery. But advances in ambulatory care now mean that many gynecologic disorders can be treated and diagnosed via a laparoscope. Laparoscopy is the visualization of the pelvic or abdominal contents via a lighted instrument (laparoscope) inserted through the abdominal wall. For gynecologic surgery, the laparoscope is usually inserted through a small incision just below the umbilicus. Additional incisions are sometimes made for the introduction of other equipment such as a laser. Gas is diffused into the abdomen; this allows better visualization of the internal structures. This pneumoperitoneum puts pressure on the diaphragm, which sometimes causes pain that is referred to the shoulder(s). The patient is usually in a lithotomy and trendelenburg (head down) position, because this displaces the abdominal contents and affords the surgeon a better view of the pelvic structures.

- Diagnostic purposes: Laparoscopy is helpful in the diagnosis of a number of gynecologic disorders, including infertility, endometriosis, ovarian cysts, pelvic pain and ectopic pregnancy.

- Therapeutic purposes: Treatment of many gynecologic disorders is possible through the laparoscope, especially with use of the laser. Treatment may include such procedures as lysis (breaking up) of adhesions and drainage of cysts. Chronic pelvic pain may be relieved by a presacral neurectomy.

- Typical procedures: Tubal ligation, lysis of adhesions, destruction of endometriomas (associated with endometriosis), biopsy, treatment of ectopic pregnancy, drainage of ovarian cysts. May also include in vitro fertilization or other fertility procedures.

- Common potential complications: Some of the potential risks of laparoscopy include damage to internal structures such as the bladder, bowel, or blood vessels with subsequent hemorrhage or infection, air embolism from the gas infusion, and cardiovascular and/or respiratory compromise from trendelenburg positioning. The potential for nerve damage in the legs exists whenever an anesthetized patient is placed in a lithotomy position. Pregnant patients are at higher risk for aspiration than non-pregnant patients.

## Intra-uterine procedures

Assessment of the uterine cavity may be undertaken to evaluate or diagnose disorders of structure or function; a number of therapeutic procedures are also performed at the same time.

- Diagnostic purposes: The inside of the uterine cavity may be explored in search of causes of abnormal bleeding or infertility. Tissue samples of the lining of the uterus, which is called the endometrium, may be secured.

- Therapeutic purposes: Scraping away the uterine lining (curretage) is performed to reduce or eliminate dysfunctional uterine bleeding (DUB), to remove nonviable products of conception after a miscarriage, or to terminate pregnancy. Retrieval of intrauterine devices and ablation of the endometrium for DUB are two other examples of therapeutic procedures.

- Typical procedures: D & C, hysteroscopy, endometrial ablation, abortion. Dye may be injected and radiographs taken during hysteroscopy to check for tubal patency as a part of a fertility assessment.

- Common potential complications: Perforation of the uterus is possible but not always serious, although hemorrhage can result. Infection is possible and can be serious. During some intra-uterine procedures such as endometrial ablation, fluids are infused into the uterus to flush it out during the procedure. These fluids can be absorbed systemically and cause a serious fluid and electrolyte imbalance or embolism.

## Cervical and vaginal procedures

Many cervical and vaginal procedures can be performed in the physician's office; those that come to the ambulatory unit often require equipment (such as a laser) that a gynecologist does not have or involve patients who are unable to tolerate the procedure in their doctor's office.

- Diagnostic purposes: Tissue samples from the vagina and cervix may be obtained for evaluation of neoplasm and other studies.

- Therapeutic purposes: Lesions, pathologic growths, and the uterus may be removed through the vagina. In pregnant patients with an incompetent cervix, a suture (cerclage) may be placed into the cervix during the first or second trimester to help preserve the pregnancy.

- Typical procedures: Cervical conization, cervical cerclage, excision of condyloma (venereal lesions), vaginal biopsy.

- Common potential complications: Complications are rare, but may be associated with laser use. The potential for bleeding and infection always exists.

## Genitalia

A number of relatively minor gynecologic procedures are performed in the physician's office or the ambulatory unit. Procedures on the external genitalia include destruction of lesions associated with sexually transmitted diseases and drainage of lesions or cysts.

- Diagnostic purposes: Most disorders of the external genitalia are evident upon observation, so there is little need for diagnosis at this point, although occasionally the physician will excise a tissue sample for pathologic evaluation.

- Therapeutic purposes: Treatment of conditions of the genitalia such as genital warts or abcesses with the use of the laser or as a minor surgical procedure.

- Typical procedures: Laser vaporization of lesions, hymenectomy or hymenotomy, marsupialization of Bartholin's cyst.

- Common potential complications: Complications are rare, but may include infection or be associated with laser use.

## Nursing strategies for the gynecologic patient

Common nursing concerns are listed in Table 12-1, Potential Nursing Diagnoses and Interventions for the Gynecologic Patient. Below, and after each specialty section, are listed common basic nursing strategies for the ambulatory gynecologic surgery patient and the rationale behind each. This is by no means an exhaustive list; detailed information about nursing care can be found in a surgical nursing textbook and other resources. Your interventions should be within the scope of your institution's practice guidelines, consistent your state's Nurse Practice Act and your license, and commensurate with your skills and training.

- Maintain the patient's privacy and dignity at all times during the perioperative period of gynecologic surgery. Remember that what is routine for the staff is not routine for the patient; unnecessary exposure and public conversation about her gynecologic disorders can increase the patient's anxiety.

### Table 12-1
### Potential Nursing Diagnoses and Interventions for the Gynecologic Patient

| Nursing Diagnosis | Sample nursing interventions |
| --- | --- |
| Injury, potential related to surgical positioning | Have two people present so the patient's legs can be raised and lowered simultaneously from the lithotomy position because this helps relieve joint strain. Pad pressure points; have stirrups at equal height, make certain patient's hands are out of the way when restoring the foot of the OR table after the procedure. |
| Infection, potential related to surgery | Wash hands before and after touching patient, teach patient principles of good hygiene. Observe principles of asepsis in the OR. Teach patient signs and symptoms of postoperative infection and instruct to call MD if noted. |
| Sexual dysfunction related to altered body structure or function | Provide privacy and nonjudgmental atmosphere in order to allow the patient to express her concerns and fears about impending gynecologic surgery. Teach her and her partner about anticipated limitations postoperatively and the reason for them. Offer emotional support to women who feel their sexuality is threatened by gynecologic procedures. |
| Self-esteem disturbance | Establish an accepting and private environment where the patient can express her concerns about impending surgery because some women view gynecologic surgery as a threat to their femininity and their identity. |
| Knowledge deficit related to lack of exposure (to ambulatory care) | Use simple diagrams when appropriate to help the patient understand her body and the procedure. Give clear concise explanations, using terminology appropriate to level of understanding; provide written information as appropriate. Orient patient to the expected events during care. Encourage patient and support person to ask questions when they do not understand anything that is happening. |
| Anxiety related to situational crisis (gynecologic surgery) | Speak softly and protect confidentiality, provide privacy, maintain patient's dignity. Avoid exposing the patient unnecessarily; keep the OR door closed, pull drapes around patient when you must check her postop. |
| Pain related to surgery | Determine nature of pain, administer analgesics as ordered; assist her to assume a more comfortable position; provide a quiet environment. |
| Grieving, anticipatory related to potential loss (ex: D & C for incomplete abortion) | Allow patient to express concerns, do not minimize or negate feelings. Ask what you or support person can do to help (ex: hold hand, hug, sit quietly with patient). Encourage expression of feelings. Refer the patient to appropriate resources or counseling for aftercare if indicated. |

Please note this is a sample of potential nursing diagnoses and is not presented as, nor intended to be, a complete care plan for the ambulatory patient. More complete information can be found in a medical surgical nursing course and textbook.

Adapted from: *Nursing Diagnosis Reference Manual* by Sheila Sparks and Cynthia M. Taylor, Springhouse Corporation, 1991, and *Overview of Anesthesia for Nurses* by L. Chitwood, Western Schools, 1992.

- Explain to women undergoing laparoscopy that postoperative shoulder pain is usually due to the gas insufflation during the procedure. Tell her the discomfort should resolve a day or two; she should notify her doctor if it does not.

- Explain "pelvic rest" to the patient for whom it is ordered after gynecologic surgery. Pelvic rest generally means not inserting anything into the vagina: no douching, tampons, or intercourse until cleared by their doctor. This aids healing after the surgery and may reduce the risk of infection.

- Notify the surgeon if the patient coming for tubal ligation (sterility) indicates that she is not certain she wishes to be rendered permanently infertile. Occasionally a patient will admit that she thought this procedure could be reversed if she subsequently changed her mind.

- Apply basic principles of body mechanics when positioning patients for gynecologic surgery; this reduces the chance of injury. The lithotomy position can result in nerve damage; placement of the legs in and out of the stirrups can result in joint and ligament strain of the back.

- Monitor the amount and type of irrigating solution if used in gynecologic surgery and inform the surgeon and anesthetist, because absorption can occur with subsequent disruption of the patient's fluid and electrolyte balance.

- Know how to secure blood products and emergency drugs should a serious or life-threatening complication occur during gynecologic surgery; this will save valuable time in the event of an emergency. While complications are rare during gynecologic surgery, injury to major internal structures or vessels is possible and shock or cardiac arrest may follow.

- Offer emotional support to the woman undergoing gynecologic surgery, because some women will feel their femininity and sexuality are threatened by such procedures.

- Tell the patient to count the number of sanitary pads used and call the doctor as instructed or if vaginal bleeding exceeds that which would normally occur during a period. Counting pads as soaked, 1/2 soaked, etc. helps estimate the amount of bleeding; bleeding heavier than a menstrual cycle generally needs to be reported to the MD. In some cases the physician may want the patient to save the pads for inspection.

# ORTHOPEDICS AND PODIATRY

Orthopedic and podiatric (foot) procedures are well represented in the ambulatory field. Many of these procedures, especially podiatry and hand or wrist surgeries, can be done under local anesthesia alone, local anesthesia with intravenous sedation, or nerve blocks. A number of podiatric surgical procedures are done in the podiatrist's office with simply local anesthesia (LA). However, a substantial number of orthopedic surgical procedures performed on the extremities, especially the lower extremities, are done under general anesthesia. Challenges to patients generally involve issues of mobility and infection.

Orthopedic and podiatric surgery are frequently performed with the use of a pneumatic tourniquet (TQ) above the operative site. This restricts blood flow and gives the surgeon a nearly bloodless field in which to work. Experts differ on the length of time this tourniquet may be left inflated, but most feel that 2 hours is about the limit. Neurovascular compromise and neuropathy can occur if the TQ is left inflated too long. Thigh TQs, used for knee surgery, are not tolerated under merely local anesthesia, or even with intravenous sedation. Patients often tolerate an ankle or upper arm TQ well in association with regional anesthesia and sedation, but once developed, tourniquet pain is severe and is only relieved by releasing the TQ or administering general anesthesia. Hypertension accompanies the development of TQ pain; it can be severe and may require treatment with intravenous (IV) antihypertensives. Most surgeons try to work quickly enough to avoid this or they halt the surgery and release the TQ for 10-20 minutes, then resume the surgery.

## Arthroscopic procedures

Just as the laparoscope revolutionized gynecologic surgery, so has the arthroscope changed the nature of orthopedic surgery. Procedures that in the past required an incision of the joint and days in the hospital now are done on an ambulatory basis. Patient recovery and return to previous levels of mobility is also usually enhanced. Arthrotomy, or incision of the joint, is still generally performed on an inpatient basis because of the need for analgesia and skilled nursing care postoperatively.

- Diagnostic purposes: Fortunately, magnetic resonance imaging (MRI) and other non-invasive techniques reduce the need for diagnostic arthroscopy. However, definitive diagnosis sometimes can't be made without direct visualization through the arthroscope, or without tissue and fluid samples.

- Therapeutic purposes: Many common joint disorders can be treated effectively with the arthroscope, which can be used for surgical techniques such as reconstruction and repair of damaged tissue. For example, torn and scarred cartilage in the knee joint can be cut and shaved away. The arthroscope may be used on other joints such as shoulders, wrist and ankles.

- Typical procedures: Arthroscopy is often associated with repairs, reconstructions, revisions, excisions, shaving, and manipulation of the joint.

- Common potential complications: Neurovascular compromise may be a concern if a pneumatic tourniquet is used. Bleeding and infection are rare but remain potential complications of arthroscopy.

**Other orthopedic and podiatric procedures.** The ambulatory care nurse will see patients with all types of orthopedic conditions, from broken bones to foreign bodies to arthritis. Patients sometimes come to ambulatory surgery for the removal of orthopedic hardware placed in a previous procedure. Other orthopedic procedures involve soft tissue, such as tendon repairs, excision of ganglion cysts and other growths, and complex joint replacements, usually in the hands or toes.

## Nursing strategies for the orthopedic patient

Common nursing concerns are listed in Table 12-2, Potential Nursing Diagnoses and Interventions for the Orthopedic Patient. Below are listed common basic nursing strategies for the ambulatory orthopedic surgery patient and the rationale behind each. This is by no means an exhaustive list; detailed information about nursing care can be found in a surgical nursing textbook and other resources.

- Assist the anesthetist in keeping the patient warm during surgery, because orthopedic surgeons working through an arthroscope usually want the OR quite cool. The cool temperature reduces fogging of the lens and enhances their comfort under surgical attire, but it can cause hypothermia in the patient. Patients undergoing GA are at greatest risk. Specially designed warming blankets and warmed fluids can help the patient's temperature remain stable. Hypothermia increases oxygen consumption, is

### Table 12-2
### Potential Nursing Diagnoses and Interventions for the Orthopedic Patient

| Nursing Diagnosis | Sample nursing interventions |
|---|---|
| Injury, potential related to sensory or motor deficits | After regional anesthesia, local anesthesia or nerve blocks, protect the affected extremity and keep it in alignment to prevent injury. Check the circulatory status of toes or fingers after application of a cast, notify MD of any changes indicating possible disruption of the neuro or vascular system. Teach cast care to patient and support person. In OR, monitor TQ time and inform the surgeon at 60 minutes, then as requested or every 15 min. thereafter. |
| Infection, potential related to surgery | Observe principles of asepsis in the OR. Teach patient signs and symptoms of postoperative infection and instruct to call MD if noted. Administer antibiotics as ordered; begin infusion in sufficient time to have all medication in by the time the TQ is inflated; this helps insure adequate circulation of the drug to all tissue. |
| Mobility impairment related to neuromuscular impairment or pain | Identify preoperative level of mobility and build upon that; when possible, have patient practice crutch walking preop; teach about preparing home environment to reduce chance of fall postop. Instruct in postop exercises as indicated, refer to Physical Therapist if ordered. Administer pain medication as ordered. Have more than one staff member present to assist the patient in getting out of bed the first time when the lower extremities are affected. |
| Knowledge deficit related to lack of exposure (to ambulatory care) | Orient patient to the expected events during care. Encourage patient and support person to ask questions when they do not understand anything that is happening. Give clear concise explanations, using terminology appropriate to level of understanding; provide written information as appropriate. Use simple diagrams when appropriate to help the patient understand his or her body and the procedure. |
| Pain related to surgery | Determine nature of pain, administer analgesics as ordered; assist to assume a more comfortable position; provide a quiet environment and distraction. If acceptable to surgeon, apply ice and elevate affected extremity. This reduces pain and swelling. |

Please note this is a sample of potential nursing diagnoses and is not presented as, nor intended to be, a complete care plan for the ambulatory patient. More complete information can be found in a medical surgical nursing course and textbook.

Adapted from: *Nursing Diagnosis Reference Manual* by Sheila Sparks and Cynthia M. Taylor, Springhouse Corporation, 1991, and *Overview of Anesthesia* for Nurses by L. Chitwood, Western Schools, 1992.

comfortable for the patient, and may prolong recovery.

- Ask the patient to indicate on which extremity the surgeon is to operate; verify this against the chart and consent. Notify the perioperative team members if there is any question and do not proceed until this issue is resolved. Going solely by the chart can lead to errors, because it could be marked incorrectly always check with the patient. Meticulous attention to this detail is essential to prevent grave errors. This can be especially true when the patient is going to be turned prone for the procedure.

- Follow the surgeon's orders after surgery on the upper or lower extremities, but note that in general orthopedic and podiatric patients do best postoperatively when the affected extremity is elevated above the level of their heart when they are recumbent. This reduces swelling, which reduces pain and enhances healing. Elevation must begin immediately postoperatively because swelling is difficult to reduce once developed.

- Apply ice packs or automatic cooling devices as ordered to reduce postoperative swelling. Monitor the skin under the ice pack to insure that the temperature is not too cold. Monitor automatic cooling devices also as they can malfunction.

- Teach the patient and support person about application of ice and elevation of the extremity if it is consistent with the physician's orders. Teach cast care and care of other orthopedic devices such as slings or braces, and give written instructions to the patient and support person to take home with them. This will help them continue appropriate care at home.

- Note that the anti-inflammatory ketorolac (Toradol) is popular in orthopedic and podiatric surgery for postop analgesia. Administer it when ordered in order to achieve maximum analgesia when needed.

- Be aware that a patient who complains of ringing in the ears (tinnitus), a funny taste in the mouth, or a feeling of doom or the "jitters" shortly after termination of IV regional anesthesia may be experiencing symptoms of an impending seizure. Notify the anesthetist and have oxygen and suction available.

- Remind the patient and support person to assess the living quarters for any possible hazards to the mobility-impaired patient. These threats include extension cords and throw rugs, pets underfoot, and toys. Clearing these hazards can prevent serious injury.

# PLASTIC SURGERY

Plastic surgery is frequently performed on an ambulatory basis; a number of freestanding ambulatory patient care facilities specialize in plastic surgery. Plastic surgery may be purely for aesthetic (cosmetic) reasons, or it may be for reconstruction after disease or trauma, or correction of congenital or acquired anomalies. Many plastic procedures are performed after local anesthesia is injected by the surgeon. Others are supplemented with IV sedation by an anesthetist or in some cases by the nurse, especially if the procedure is expected to last more than 1-2 hours. On other occasions, general anesthesia is necessary. This is often the case in breast surgery, including reductions or augmentations.

## Reconstruction, revision, excision, and aesthetic procedures

Plastic surgery procedures in this category may range from a simple excision of a skin lesion to a complex skin graft.

- Diagnostic purposes: Plastic surgeons commonly remove lesions on the face or neck for examination and diagnosis of pathology. Small lesions are usually removed under local anesthesia.

- Therapeutic purposes: Plastic surgery is a part of the treatment of a number of disorders. Reconstruction or revision procedures are performed after illness or injury such as congenital malformations, cancer treatment, burns, and other trauma. Reconstructive breast surgery may follow mastectomy; breast reduction often frees large-breasted women from back, neck and shoulder pain.

- Typical procedures: Excision of lesions, breast reduction, augmentation (implants), or mastopexy (revision of pendulous breasts), rhinoplasty (nose), blepharoplasty (eye), rhytidectomy (face lift), submental (neck), lipectomy (fat removal, usually by suction), tatoo removal and laser treatment of certain skin disorders, skin grafts, placement of tissue expanders after trauma or extensive surgery.

- Common potential complications: Plastic surgery is quite safe when performed by qualified surgeons. However, because large amounts of local anesthetics are often used, toxicity can develop, especially when epinephrine is also injected. Since these patients are often covered with surgical drapes, changes in the patient's respirations or color may be masked. Retching and coughing postop are to be avoided because of the potential tension on sutures. Postoperative bleeding and swelling can distort the incision and affect the final results. Suction lipectomy has been associated with major fluid shifts in the body; electrolyte imbalance, hypotension, and edema may result. Most nurses are also by now aware of the controversies surrounding silicone-filled breast implants, which are no longer in general use.

### Nursing strategies for the plastic surgery patient

Common nursing concerns are listed in Table 12-3, Potential Nursing Diagnoses and Interventions for the Plastic Surgery Patient. Below are listed common basic nursing strategies for the ambulatory plastic surgery patient and the rationale behind each. This is by no means an exhaustive list; detailed information about nursing care can be found in a surgical nursing textbook and other resources.

- Advise smokers to quit; smoking cessation will promote health and aid healing by eliminating the vasoconstrictive effects of nicotine. Advise the patient that smoking contributes to the development of facial wrinkles.

- Know your responsibilities and limitations if you are asked to administer IV sedation while a plastic surgeon works. Serious patient injury or death and professional liability could result from administering conscious sedation; check your facility's policy and your state's nurse practice act; refer to Appendix B.

- Maintain voice contact and leave one of the patient's hands exposed when the plastic surgery patient will be covered with surgical drapes. This will help you monitor the patient's condition and level of consciousness.

- Set your own feelings aside when caring for the plastic surgery patient. Regardless of your personal feelings about aesthetic surgery, the patient is entitled to your full and best care.

# OTOLARYNGOLOGY & ORAL SURGERY

Otolaryngology (ear, nose or throatENT) and dental procedures are well represented in ambulatory surgery, especially in pediatrics. The care of these patients can be especially challenging because manipulation of the airway may be involved. A number of ENT procedures such as septoplasty can be performed with local anesthesia (LA), but many require general anesthesia. This LA usually contains epinephrine which constricts blood vessels to reduce bleeding in the surgical field; cocaine is often used

### Table 12-3
### Potential Nursing Diagnoses and Interventions for the Plastic Surgery Patient

| Nursing Diagnosis | Sample nursing interventions |
| --- | --- |
| Fluid volume deficit or excess | Note that suction lipectomy can result in shifts of extracellular and intravascular fluids; the patient may become hypovolemic or edematous from fluid overload. Monitor fluids carefully and inform surgeon of the amount of material suctioned at regular intervals. Some experts recommend no more than 1500 ml maximum to be removed at one time, but this must be adapted to the patient's condition and size. |
| Infection, potential related to surgery | Observe principles of asepsis in the OR. Teach patient signs and symptoms of postoperative infection and instruct to call MD if noted. |
| Body image disturbance | Accept patient's perception of self and offer opportunity to express feelings. Refer patient to counselor or community resource like a support group of people with similar concerns (ex: burns). Offer positive reinforcement of patient's efforts at adaptation. |
| Self-esteem disturbance | Preoperatively, encourage patient to express feelings and to examine motives for and expectation from aesthetic plastic surgery. This will help him or her to define concerns and expectations more clearly. Set your own feelings aside and offer non-judgmental support of the aesthetic plastic surgery patient during the perioperative period. |
| Pain related to surgery | Determine nature of pain, administer analgesics as ordered; assist to assume a more comfortable position; provide a quiet environment and distraction. If acceptable to surgeon, apply ice or elevate affected area. This reduces pain and swelling. |

Please note this is a sample of potential nursing diagnoses and is not presented as, nor intended to be, a complete care plan for the ambulatory patient. More complete information can be found in a medical surgical nursing course and textbook.

Adapted from: *Nursing Diagnosis Reference Manual* by Sheila Sparks and Cynthia M. Taylor, Springhouse Corporation, 1991, and *Overview of Anesthesia* for Nurses by L. Chitwood, Western Schools, 1992.

for the same reason. Patients receiving general anesthesia are usually intubated to allow control of the airway because the anesthetist will move away from the head of the bed in the OR in order to allow surgical access. Postoperative nausea and vomiting (N & V) are relatively common because of blood loss down the throat and into the stomach or equilibrium disturbances after ear procedures. Common ambulatory ENT procedures are reviewed below; pediatric ENT surgery is discussed in Chapter 11.

### Ear procedures

Many ear procedures are performed on an ambulatory basis; these include plastic revisions such as otoplasty as well as reconstruction, biopsy, revision, excision, and incision.

- Diagnostic purposes: Tissue biopsies may be taken from growths or other lesions.

- Therapeutic purposes: Ear procedures are commonly performed to enhance hearing or appearance, reduce infections, correct pathology, drain fluid, retrieve foreign bodies, and correct or reduce hearing disorders.

- Typical procedures: Myringotomy, stapedectomy, mastoidectomy, tympanoplasty, otoplasty.

- Common potential complications: Nausea and vomiting, dizziness, and vertigo may occur postoperatively. There may be bleeding or infection if an incision was made. If a microscope is used, the patient must be still in order to avoid injury; the nurse should insure that the microscope has an emergency stop to prevent patient injury.

## Nose and sinus procedures

Surgical procedures on the nose and sinuses are commonly performed in the ambulatory unit. Surgeons often prefer LA to GA because intraoperative bleeding is generally reduced by the addition of epinephrine to the LA.

- Diagnostic purposes: Polyps and tissue may be excised for biopsy.

- Therapeutic purposes: Surgical intervention of nasal or sinus pathology generally revolves around clearing the airway to facilitate air passage and reduce pain from pathology.

- Typical procedures: Endoscopic sinus surgery, septoplasty and rhinoplasty, polyp removal, submucous resection, treatment of epistaxis.

- Common potential complications: Surgical manipulation of the nose and upper airway can lead to bleeding, swelling of tissue, and airway obstruction. Airway obstruction leads to death in a matter of minutes. For this reason, patients who were intubated during surgery are generally not extubated after surgery until they are awake, with protective gag and swallowing reflexes intact. Waiting until the patient is awake to extubate helps insure that he or she will be able to maintain ventilation; waiting until the return of protective reflexes helps insure that the patient will be able to protect the airway from drainage or secretions. Bleeding after upper airway surgery can be intense; infection is always possible.

## Throat procedures

Surgical manipulation of the airway including the mouth and throat structures is commonly performed on an ambulatory basis. Major surgery such as laryngectomy is still limited to hospitalized patients, though many are seen on the morning of surgery and prepared for the surgery by the ambulatory staff of hospitals.

- Diagnostic purposes: Tissue samples may be taken for pathologic examination; laryngoscopy may be performed in the ambulatory surgical setting to directly visualize the vocal cords and diagnose pathology.

- Therapeutic purposes: Procedures on the throat and mouth are generally performed to reduce airway obstruction (as in snoring), and to correct pathology.

- Typical procedures: Adenoidectomy, tonsillectomy, laryngoscopy, teflon injection of vocal cords, biopsy, fracture repair of mandible.

- Common potential complications: The same precautions listed above about possible airway obstruction and bleeding apply to procedures on the mouth and throat. While most of these procedures are completed without incident, complications can be swift and fatal. Dental injury is possible whenever surgical instruments and airway manipulation equipment are inserted into the mouth.

## Oral surgery

Many oral surgeons perform surgical procedures such as the extraction of wisdom teeth in their offices. Intravenous access is usually secured, and the oral surgeon or assistant may administer sedation. Some oral surgeons bring patients to an ambulatory OR for more complex procedures.

- Diagnostic purposes: Most diagnoses have already been made by the time a patient undergoes oral surgery, but biopsies or tissue samples are occasionally secured.

- Therapeutic purposes: Oral surgery procedures often involve reconstructive or restorative surgeries.

- Typical procedures: Extraction of wisdom and other teeth, fracture repair of mandible, placement of wires, hardware, and protheses.

- Common potential complications: The same precautions listed above about possible airway obstruction and bleeding apply to oral surgery. While most of these procedures are completed without incident, complications can be swift and fatal. Close monitoring is essential. Many oral surgery patients often have packing in place; this could obstruct the airway in the somnolent patient. Patients discharged with packing in place must be aware of its presence and how to remove it if necessary or how to apply fresh packing if indicated.

## Nursing strategies for the ENT patient

Common nursing concerns are listed in Table 12-4, Potential Nursing Diagnoses and Interventions for the ENT Patient. Below are listed common basic nursing strategies for the ambulatory ENT surgery patient and the rationale behind each. This is by no means an exhaustive list; detailed information about nursing care can be found in a surgical nursing textbook and other resources.

- Be aware that the postop ENT or oral surgery patient who complains of having to swallow frequently may be having significant bleeding. Assess the patient and notify the surgeon of the patient's complaint and the results of your assessment. Early identification of postop bleeding can prevent disaster.

- Tell the patient to avoid blowing the nose after nose surgery, if this is consistent with the doctor's orders. This can reduce the chance of postoperative bleeding.

- Note that epinephrine and cocaine used during surgery may stimulate the cardiovascular system; cardiac arrhythmias and cardiovascular collapse may result. Know the location of emergency resuscitation drugs before beginning a case; this can help save precious time in the event of an emergency.

- Keep in mind that surgical manipulation of the airway passages can compromise the airway. Be prepared to secure emergency supplies, call for help, and assist other team members should airway difficulties arise. Proper planning saves valuable minutes and increases the nurse's confidence in delivering care.

- Elevate the head of the patient's bed after surgery if acceptable to the surgeon. Apply ice if ordered. This reduces swelling and pain and also helps ease the patient's breathing.

- Check the security of the position of the microscope if one is used in surgery. An unsecure microscope could fall onto the patient, causing injury.

- Notify the surgeon immediately when a patient who has had endoscopic sinus surgery complains

### Table 12-4
### Potential Nursing Diagnoses and Interventions for the ENT or Oral Surgery Patient

| Nursing Diagnosis | Sample nursing interventions |
| --- | --- |
| Airway clearance, ineffective related to obstruction or secretions | Have suction and oxygen available at patient's bedside; monitor respiratory status and ventilatory exchange; elevate head of bed; administer warm moist oxygen by mask or face tent (if consistent with physician's orders); provide tissues and emesis basin for patient comfort. Know the location of emergency airway equipment; notify surgeon/anesthetist of any concerns regarding airway. |
| Infection, potential related to surgery | Observe principles of asepsis in the OR. Teach patient signs and symptoms of postoperative infection and instruct to call MD if noted. |
| Body image disturbance | Be aware that bandages, swelling, and discoloration may distress patient. Allow patient to express concerns; accentuate the positive, including enhanced appearance or resolution of pathology. |
| Tissue perfusion alteration related to hypovolemia | Monitor vital signs until stable and then at regular intervals, evaluate for bleeding; administer fluids as ordered. Maintain intravenous access until all potential for bleeding has passed. |
| Pain related to surgery | Determine nature of pain, administer analgesics as ordered; assist to assume a more comfortable position; provide a quiet environment and distraction. If acceptable to surgeon, apply ice to affected area. This reduces pain and swelling. |

Please note this is a sample of potential nursing diagnoses and is not presented as, nor intended to be, a complete care plan for the ambulatory patient. More complete information can be found in a medical surgical nursing course and textbook.

Adapted from: *Nursing Diagnosis Reference Manual* by Sheila Sparks and Cynthia M. Taylor, Springhouse Corporation, 1991, and *Overview of Anesthesia* for Nurses by L. Chitwood, Western Schools, 1992.

---

of visual disturbance or you note clear fluid coming from the patient's nose. The former could be related to damage to the optic structures; the latter could be a leak of cerebrospinal fluid (CSF). Both of these are serious complications; early intervention can mean the difference in outcome.

- Remember that tonsillectomies and other brief airway procedures, while common and routine in the ambulatory unit, have the potential for serious bleeding and airway obstruction. These patients require skilled perioperative nursing care until it has been determined that the airway is patent and all bleeding has stopped. Otherwise, patient death may result.

- Follow your facility's guidelines on extubating patients after ENT surgery, because airway closure or obstruction after extubation might result. If in doubt, it is generally safer to leave the endotracheal tube in place until the patient is evaluated by the anesthetist. This is because complications from leaving an endotracheal tube in place too long are usually less serious and more easily rectified than complications from taking it out too soon.

- Apply a mask of warm humidified oxygen after surgery if the surgeon agrees. Humidified air can reduce pain.

# UROLOGIC SURGERY

Endoscopes also moved many urologic procedures into the ambulatory arena. Urologic patients are often children (see Chapter 11), or adult males. Urologic procedures may be diagnostic or therapeutic. Some procedures are done under local anesthesia; others require GA or RA.

## General urologic procedures

Urologic procedures are often performed with the patient in a lithotomy or frog leg position; procedures on the scrotum usually require the patient to be supine. Access is often through the urethra rather than an incision; radiographs may be taken.

- Diagnostic purposes: Biopsy specimens from genitourinary structures may be obtained for further evaluation. Radiographs may be taken to aid in diagnosis; studies may include the kidneys.

- Therapeutic purposes: Urologic procedures may involve elective procedures such as vasectomy or vasectomy reversal, or palliative or curative procedures such as cancer treatments.

- Typical procedures: Cystoscopy, placement of stents, vasectomy or reversal, bladder or prostate biopsy, circumcision, orchiopexy, nephrostomy, urethral dilation. Burden (1993) reports that some ambulatory facilities are performing transurethral resection of the prostate (TURP).

- Common potential complications: The potential exists for the patient to acquire a urinary tract infection before leaving the ambulatory care unit, so strict attention to asepsis is essential. While some bleeding is to be expected, frank hemorrhage can result. Patients may also complain of urinary retention and inability to void. Rarely, the bladder or ureters can be perforated. The TURP procedure involves use of irrigating solutions that may be absorbed systemically, causing serious disruptions of fluid and electrolyte balance.

## Lithotripsy

In the 1980s, a method of pulverizing kidney stones with shock waves was developed; this reduced the need for major surgery that required opening the flank and exploring for the stone which is often trapped in the ureter. High-energy shock waves break the stone into small pieces that can then be passed in the urine. This is called extracorporeal shock-wave lithotripsy (ESWL). The patient is immersed in a bath of water, the stone's location is verified, and then one to two thousand bursts of shock waves are directed at it. Some patients receive epidural anesthesia (because of the practical difficulty of administering GA to a patient sitting in water and removed from the anesthetist); many patients receive only conscious sedation. Potential complications include hypothermia and other changes in vital signs from immersion in the water.

## Nursing strategies for the urologic surgery patient.

Common nursing concerns are listed in Table 12-5, Potential Nursing Diagnoses and Interventions for the Urology Patient. Below are listed common basic nursing strategies for the ambulatory urologic surgery patient and the rationale behind each. This is by no means an exhaustive list; detailed information about nursing care can be found in a surgical nursing textbook and other resources. Note that some of the

### Table 12-5
### Potential Nursing Diagnoses and Interventions for the Urologic Patient

| Nursing Diagnosis | Sample nursing interventions |
| --- | --- |
| Urinary elimination pattern alteration, related to obstruction | When allowed and the patient is stable, transport to bathroom and provide privacy for voiding, assist male patient to stand to void. Offer warm beverage such as tea; run water. |
| Infection, potential related to surgery | Avoid reflux of urine from collection bag back into bladder. Observe principles of asepsis in the OR. Teach patient signs and symptoms of postoperative infection and instruct to call MD if noted. |
| Sexual dysfunction related to altered body structure or function | Provide privacy and nonjudgmental atmosphere in order to allow the patient to express his or her concerns and fears about urologic surgery. Teach partners about anticipated limitations postoperatively and the reason for them. Offer emotional support to patients who feel their sexuality is threatened by urologic surgery. |
| Pain related to surgery | Determine nature of pain, administer analgesics as ordered; assist to assume a more comfortable position; provide a quiet environment and distraction. |

Please note this is a sample of potential nursing diagnoses and is not presented as, nor intended to be, a complete care plan for the ambulatory patient. More complete information can be found in a medical surgical nursing course and textbook.

Adapted from: *Nursing Diagnosis Reference Manual* by Sheila Sparks and Cynthia M. Taylor, Springhouse Corporation, 1991, and *Overview of Anesthesia* for Nurses by L. Chitwood, Western Schools, 1992.

---

strategies for urology patients will overlap with those for gynecologic patients.

- Explain to the urologic patient that some blood in the urine is common for a day or two after surgery. Follow the doctor's orders, or advise the patient to consult his or her physician if the bleeding becomes bright red or is associated with abdominal or pelvic pain and/or a fever. These instructions help reduce the patient's anxiety and guide him or her to appropriate follow-up care.

- Palpate gently the abdomen for any signs of a distended bladder; notify the surgeon if the patient is unable to void after standard nursing measures such as providing privacy or running water have failed.

- Encourage po fluids if ordered to maintain adequate hydration and urine flow.

- Remind ESWL patients to strain their urine and save stone fragments for their doctor if ordered. This helps the physician evaluate the results of the treatment.

- Provide privacy and maintain the patient's dignity, because unnecessary exposure during urologic procedures can distress the patient.

- Wash hands before and after caring for the patient, because this will reduce the incidence of infection postop. Teach patient importance of handwashing at home.

- Note that most ambulatory facilities require the patient to void spontaneously before discharge; notify the physician if this is the case and the patient is unable to void.

# OPHTHALMIC SURGERY

Ophthalmic surgery is one of the most commonly performed ambulatory surgical procedures. Patients are frequently quite young (see Chapter 11) or quite old (cataract surgery). Ophthalmologic surgery is well suited to ambulatory care because it is often performed under local anesthesia (LA) with conscious sedation. In many cases, the ophthalmologist administers this LA in the form of a retrobulbar block, which consists of injections around the eye globe. This may be done in the preoperative preparation area or in the OR. Present to assist the ophthalmologist and administer sedation during this time is a nurse, and often an anesthetist. In some situations, the anesthetist will perform this block. Ophthalmic surgeons also commonly apply topical anesthetics to the eye. Two classifications of ophthalmic surgical procedures, intraocular and extraocular, are discussed below. Because these procedures are seldom diagnostic, only typical procedures and common complications are discussed.

## Extraocular procedures

This refers to surgical procedures on structures outside of the globe itself.

- Typical procedures: Surgery on the muscles connected to the eye such as strabismus, lacrimal duct probing, lid procedures, and removal of the eye (enucleation).

- Common potential complications: The oculocardiac reflex occurs from pressure on the globe or the traction on the structures around it and may develop at any time during the procedure. This can result in sudden and severe bradycardia or even asystole. The patient requires continuous heart rate monitoring during ophthalmic surgery, and atropine should be readily available for injection, although the heart rate usually returns to normal when the stimulus (such as pressing on the globe) stops. Many professionals believe all ophthalmic surgery patients should have intravenous access established in case these complications develop. Injection of retrobulbar anesthesia has been complicated by apparent inadvertent injection into the CSF with resulting cardiovascular collapse (Tatum & Defalque, 1994). Because the ophthalmic patient is usually covered by surgical drapes, hypoventilation and hypoxia are potential threats. Infection, as with any procedure, remains a possibility.

### Intraocular procedures

Cataract extraction is one of the most common ambulatory surgical procedures performed, but other intraocular procedures are also well suited to ambulatory care.

- Typical procedures: Cataract extraction, glaucoma surgeries, laser surgery, vitreo-retinal surgeries.

- Common potential complications: The same precautions listed above for extraocular procedures are also applicable to intraocular procedures.

### Nursing strategies for the ophthalmic surgery patient

Common nursing concerns are listed in Table 12-6, Potential Nursing Diagnoses and Interventions for

### Table 12-6
### Potential Nursing Diagnoses and Interventions for the Ophthalmic Surgery Patient

| Nursing Diagnosis | Sample nursing interventions |
|---|---|
| Decreased cardiac output as a result of electrophysiologic disorder | Monitor patient's heart rhythm during retrobulbar block and during ophthalmic surgery, in order to detect changes such as bradycardia that herald triggering of the oculcardiac reflex. If an anesthetist is not present, have available atropine and oxygen for emergency administration. |
| Infection, potential related to surgery | Observe principles of asepsis in the OR. Teach patient signs and symptoms of postoperative infection and instruct to call MD if noted. |
| Mobility impairment related to perceptual impairment & sensory alteration related to sensory deprivation | Be aware that bandages will restrict the patient's visual field and mobility. Discuss preparing a safe home environment free of obstacles and potential hazards such as cords, rugs, or other hazards. Discuss ways in which the patient's home environment can be arranged to offset deficit. Hold patient's hand when talking if appropriate; offer personal stereo headset so patient can listen to music. Reorient patient to environment frequently |
| Pain related to surgery | Determine nature of pain, administer analgesics as ordered; assist to assume a more comfortable position; provide a quiet environment and distraction. If acceptable to surgeon, apply ice to affected area. This reduces pain and swelling. |

Please note this is a sample of potential nursing diagnoses and is not presented as, nor intended to be, a complete care plan for the ambulatory patient. More complete information can be found in a medical surgical nursing course and textbook.

Adapted from: *Nursing Diagnosis Reference Manual* by Sheila Sparks and Cynthia M. Taylor, Springhouse Corporation, 1991, and *Overview of Anesthesia* for Nurses by L. Chitwood, Western Schools, 1992.

the Ophthalmic Surgery Patient. Below are listed common basic nursing strategies for the ambulatory ophthalmology patient and the rationale behind each. This is by no means an exhaustive list; detailed information about nursing care can be found in a surgical nursing textbook and other resources.

- Administer eye drops before and after surgery as ordered, because these drops facilitate the surgery and incorrect administration can reduce probability of a good outcome.

- Teach patient and support person about eye drop instillation and dressing changes at home after surgery if indicated. Give them this information in written form and allow them a chance to practice instillation under your guidance if possible. This helps increase their learning and confidence level.

- Maintain voice contact with the eye surgery patient. This is part of assessing the patient's response to surgery and any sedatives that have been administered and can alert you to changes in the level of consciousness.

- Elevate the head of the patient's bed after surgery if acceptable to the surgeon. This reduces swelling and pain and also helps ease the patient's breathing.

- Tell the patient, if consistent with the ophthalmologist's orders, that he or she should not hang the head down or bend over because this will increase intraocular pressure.

- Check the security of the position of the microscope if one is used in surgery. An unsecure microscope could fall onto the patient, causing injury.

- Announce your presence to the patient who has one or both eyes bandaged; orient the patient frequently and offer explanations of what you are doing. This can help reduce anxiety.

## CARDIOVASCULAR SURGERY

Cardiac patients even appear in the ambulatory unit. Ambulatory cardiac procedures might include cardiac biopsy after a heart transplant or implantation of a pacemaker. Principles of nursing care are generally the same as if the patient was inpatient, but the emphasis is on returning the patient to his or her home. Infection, arrhythmias, perforation, and hemorrhage may be specific concerns.

## GENERAL SURGERY

General surgeons continue to perform an increasing number of procedures on an ambulatory basis. Hernia repair is now sometimes performed with the aid of the laparoscope, as is cholecystectomy. Breast biopsy and hemorrhoidectomy are also commonly performed on an ambulatory basis. Principles of care are the same as for the hospitalized patient with the exception of preparing the patient to go home that same day.

## SUMMARY

This chapter explored many of the surgical specialties and grouped common surgical procedures into classifications. The classifications were then described in terms of diagnostic or therapeutic use. Examples of typical procedures within that classification were presented and common associated complications were discussed. Sample nursing diagnoses were proposed for each section and specific nursing strategies were presented.

## CRITICAL CONCEPTS

- Airway compromise or closure may develop after surgical manipulation of any part of the airway such as the throat.

- Sudden and severe bradycardia or asystole (oculocardiac reflex) may develop during retrobulbar block or ophthalmic surgery. It results from pressure on the eye or traction on the muscles around the eye.

- Gynecologic and urologic patients should have their privacy protected and their dignity maintained during the perioperative period.

- Nurses may need to set aside their personal feelings about some surgical procedures in order to provide the patient with non-judgmental care.

# EXAM QUESTIONS

## Chapter 12

Questions 71-85

71. A common postoperative goal for tonsillectomy patients is maintenance of a patent:

    a. foley catheter
    b. intravenous line
    c. airway
    d. intrathecal shunt

72. Elevation of the affected extremity after podiatric surgery helps reduce postoperative:

    a. pain and swelling
    b. hypotension and arrhythmias
    c. fever and malaise
    d. nausea and vomiting

73. Nerve damage in the legs would be most likely to develop as a result of which of the following surgical positions?

    a. lithotomy
    b. supine
    c. Fowler's
    d. prone

74. Impaired mobility would be a common nursing diagnosis for which class of patients?

    a. gynecologic
    b. orthopedic
    c. pediatric
    d. urologic

75. A sudden bradycardia that develops during eye surgery would most likely be due to:

    a. Hunter's syndrome
    b. oculocardiac reflex
    c. diving reflex
    d. sympathomimetic reflex

76. Common concerns of ambulatory surgery patients are:

    a. pain and complications
    b. infections and nausea
    c. postop mobility and pain
    d. surgeon's skills and the bill

77. As you prepare your patient to undergo a tubal ligation, she mentions that she expects to have the procedure reversed in a few years when she finishes school. You should further explore her understanding of tubal ligation and then:

    a. cancel the case and send her home
    b. notify her doctor
    c. ask her husband what he wants her to do
    d. send her to surgery

78. The diffusion of a gas into the abdomen during laparoscopy results in:

    a. diving reflex
    b. pneumothorax
    c. pneumoperitoneum
    d. hemathorax

79. The intrauterine infusion of irrigating solutions during endometrial ablation can cause:

    a. fluid and electrolyte imbalance
    b. hypotension
    c. pneumoperitoneum and hemorrhage
    d. diuresis

80. "Pelvic rest" is often ordered for which class of postoperative patients?

    a. orthopedic
    b. ophthalmic
    c. gynecologic
    d. neurologic

81. What do orthopedic and poediatric surgeons frequently use to reduce bleeding during surgery?

    a. cautery
    b. tourniquet
    c. silver nitrate
    d. laser

82. Which of the following may be a complication of tourniquet use?

    a. hematuria
    b. hypotension
    c. asphyxia
    d. neurovascular compromise

83. Common nursing diagnoses for orthopedic patients include:

    a. infection and mobility impairment
    b. knowledge deficit and personal identity disturbance
    c. self-care deficit and incontinence
    d. powerlessness and parental role conflict

84. Patients who had surgical procedures that involved the airway are usually extubated:

    a. awake
    b. asleep
    c. after discharge
    d. unconscious

85. Two grave complications that may develop after oral, nasal, or throat surgery are:

    a. infection and oliguria
    b. depression and bleeding
    c. bleeding and airway obstruction
    d. dental injury and infection

# CHAPTER 13

# NURSING CONSIDERATIONS IN DIAGNOSTIC AND THERAPEUTIC PROCEDURES

## CHAPTER OBJECTIVE

After completing this chapter, you should be better prepared to plan and implement nursing care for ambulatory patients undergoing common diagnostic and therapeutic procedures.

## LEARNING OBJECTIVES:

After reading this chapter, you should be able to:

1. Select potential nursing diagnoses for different classes of patients undergoing diagnostic or therapeutic procedures.

2. Identify common needs of patients undergoing routine ambulatory diagnostic and therapeutic procedures.

3. Specify nursing measures that enhance the potential for good results from the diagnostic or therapeutic procedure.

4. Identify nursing strategies for preparing ambulatory patients for diagnostic or therapeutic procedures.

5. Recognize common complications that may develop during or after ambulatory diagnostic or therapeutic procedures.

## INTRODUCTION

An incredible variety of special procedures are performed on an ambulatory basis. Many of these procedures are relatively minor and routine, such as a chest x-ray or ultrasound. Other procedures, such as cardiac catheterization, are far more hazardous but are still often performed on an ambulatory basis. In many of these cases, the ambulatory patient care nurse's role is to prepare or recover the patient, and in some cases to assist the physician or other professional in performing the procedure. But there are a number of procedures that are now even being performed by the nurse, such as instilling chemotherapeutic agents into the bladder or injecting subcutaneous abdominal implants with hormone suppressing drugs. You can expect to be involved in even more complex procedures in the future.

This chapter reviews common diagnostic and therapeutic ambulatory procedures in the following classifications: gastroenterology, radiology, cardiology, obstetrics, parenteral therapy, pulmonary, pain management, and others. Common complications and nursing strategies associated with each are reviewed. Clearly, it would be impossible to discuss or review every ambulatory diagnostic or therapeutic procedure; this chapter only serves as an overview and introduction. The chapter closes with a summary and a list of the critical concepts presented.

# DIAGNOSTIC AND THERAPEUTIC PROCEDURES

In the sections that follow, you will be presented with an overview of concerns that are common to ambulatory diagnostic and therapeutic procedures in that specialty. After a brief review of common procedures, common complications will be addressed, and then nursing strategies will be presented for patients undergoing the procedures. For each of the nursing strategy groups, you should realize that this is by no means an exhaustive list; detailed information about nursing care can be found in a medical and surgical nursing textbooks and other resources. Your interventions should always be within the scope of your institution's practice guidelines, consistent with your state's Nurse Practice Act and your license, and commensurate with your skills and training.

# GASTROINTESTINAL PROCEDURES

Many gastrointestinal (GI) procedures are performed on an ambulatory basis. The GI procedures unit may be part of a hospital, a freestanding unit, or connected with a gastroenterologist's office. The Society of Gastroenterology Nurses and Associates has developed a resource, the *Manual of Gastrointestinal Procedures,* in which you can find additional information about nursing the patient undergoing a GI procedure.

## Diagnostic procedures

GI diagnostic procedures frequently involve the use of the endoscope, a device for viewing structures in the body. The endoscope is a flexible tube that incorporates fiberoptic technology, allowing photography or videography of the internal structures during the procedure. GI diagnostic procedures often include the use of x-rays, collection of specimens such as brushings and washings, and biopsy.

**Colonoscopy.** Colonoscopy is an examination of the colon, which is the large intestine that runs from the rectum to the ileocecal valve where it joins the small intestine.

- Common indications: Evaluation of suspected or confirmed disease; visualization of internal structures; securing specimens for further testing. Also used therapeutically to decompress or dilate the colon, and cauterize bleeding sites; polypectomy refers to the removal of polyps with the endoscope.

- Complications: Perforation or puncture of the colon, hemorrhage, infection.

**Esophagogastroduodenoscopy (EGD).** Visualization of the esophagus, stomach, and proximal duodenum via the endoscope.

- Common indications: Evaluation of upper GI concerns such as dysphagia, GI bleeding, esophageal varices; specimen retrieval; cauterize bleeding sites.

- Complications: Perforation or puncture of the upper GI tract, hemorrhage, infection, aspiration.

**Flexible sigmoidoscopy.** Visualization of the sigmoid and descending colon via the endoscope. A rigid instrument is sometimes used in proctosigmoidoscopy.

- Common indications: Evaluation for abnormal conditions such as colitis and diarrhea or bleeding; screening for colorectal cancer.

- Complications: Perforation or puncture, hemorrhage.

**Endoscopic retrograde cholangiopancreatography (ERCP).** Injection of dye for radiologic visualization of the biliary and pancreatic ducts.

- Common indications: Evaluation for abnormal conditions related to the structure or function of the biliary and pancreatic ducts, such as cancer or obstruction. Also used therapeutically, as in placement of stents (thin hollow tubes) and drains

- Complications: Perforation, hemorrhage, infection, allergic reaction to contrast medium (dye), cholangitis, pancreatitis.

**Percutaneous liver biopsy.** This is a non-surgical technique to secure liver tissue.

- Common indications: Evaluation of abnormal conditions related to the structure or function of the liver such as hepatitis, jaundice, cancer.

- Complications: Damage to liver resulting in hemorrhage or infection, pneumothorax, death.

## Therapeutic procedures

Therapeutic procedures are often done in conjunction with diagnostic procedures; they are reflected in the procedures reviewed below.

**Esophageal dilatation.** If the esophagus is narrowed, swallowing food can become difficult or impossible. Dilatation of the esophagus is performed by inserting successively larger dilators until the stricture is relieved.

- Indications: Narrowing of the esophagus secondary to malignancy, radiation therapy, or scleroderma, among other conditions.

- Complications: Perforation of the esophagus, hemorrhage, aspiration.

**Electrocautery.** Electrocautery is the use of a metal instrument, heated by electricity, to burn and destroy tissue. Electrocautery is often employed to destroy lesions and halt bleeding.

- Indications: Abnormal growths in the GI tract such as polyps or other lesions; GI bleeding.

- Complications: Perforation, hemorrhage, explosion, burns.

**Sclerotherapy.** Esophageal varices are dilated veins in the esophagus that can rupture and bleed. Sclerotherapy involves injecting an agent into the varices to stop the bleeding and harden (or sclerose) the varices.

- Indications: Bleeding of esophageal varices, sometimes as a temporary intervention until surgery. Often performed in patients who are poor candidates for surgical intervention.

- Complications: Perforation, hemorrhage (may lead to death), aspiration.

**Percutaneous Endoscopic Gastrostomy (PEG).** This is placement of a feeding tube into the stomach or jejunum; it is an alternative to surgical placement of a feeding tube.

- Indications: To deliver food to the patient who no longer gets adequate nutrition from oral ingestion of food; patients at risk for aspiration (those with incompetent gag reflex).

- Complications: Perforation, hemorrhage, aspiration.

## Nursing considerations for the patient undergoing a GI procedure

Below are listed common basic nursing strategies for the ambulatory GI patient and the rationale behind each.

- Know and follow principles of safe practice when using electrocautery units, because the patient could suffer burns and other untoward effects.

- Verify consent has been signed before giving preoperative sedation, because the legality can be questioned if it is signed after sedation.

- Note that liver biopsy patients often are required to lie on their right side for several hours after the procedure because this can have a tamponade effect on any bleeding.

- Use aseptic technique as indicated to reduce the chance of spreading infection from one patient to another in the GI lab.

- Know the location of the emergency code cart and how to call for help in the event of an emergency. This can save valuable seconds in an emergency.

- Follow your institution's policy and your state's nurse practice act if you agree to administer conscious sedation for GI procedures. Advanced knowledge and skills are essential to safe administration of these drugs; see Appendix B on Conscious Sedation and Suggested Reading by Kidwell, and Murphy for more information.

- Be aware that perforation of any part of the GI tract, such as the bowel or esophagus can be a grave complication; be prepared for emergency surgery if necessary.

- Educate the patient and his or her support person in what to expect during a GI procedure, because knowing what to expect can decrease patient anxiety. Include information about positioning and sensations or noises the patient may experience during the procedure. If possible, visit the GI lab yourself and observe some common procedures; this can give you more confidence in your teaching.

- Provide reassurance and psychological support during the procedure, because this increases the patient's comfort and can reduce anxiety.

- Be certain that the patient followed any bowel preparation instructions carefully, because the procedure may have to be cancelled otherwise.

- Instruct patient and support person in aftercare, including signs and symptoms of complications. Many facilities use postprocedure instruction sheets to facilitate this transfer of information (see Figure 13-1).

- Remember that since many patients receive IV sedation during GI procedures, they must have someone drive them home because they would be considered an impaired driver otherwise.

# RADIOLOGIC PROCEDURES

Radiologic procedures can be invasive, such as an arteriogram, or non-invasive, such as a CAT scan. Radiologic procedures may be routine, such as chest

# CHAPTER 13 — NURSING CONSIDERATIONS IN DIAGNOSTIC AND THERAPEUTIC PROCEDURES

## SAINT FRANCIS HOSPITAL
### OUTPATIENT SERVICE DEPARTMENT
### FOLLOW-UP RECORD

IMPRINT THIS AREA

Date _____ Time _____ Completed  Yes _____ No _____
24hrs, 48hrs, 72hrs       2nd Call Indicated _____
Date of Surgery _____ Type of Procedure _____
                          (Patient's Description)

1. Patient able to resume ADL    Yes _____ No _____
2. Patient able to resume normal diet   Yes _____ No _____
3. Did patient get discharge prescriptions filled?  Yes _____ No _____ NA _____
   If Yes, when? _____ Any side effects experienced? _____
4. Patient experienced nausea   Yes _____ No _____ Vomiting  Yes _____ No _____
   What did patient do for relief? _____
5. Any pain experienced from surgery   Yes _____ No _____
   If Yes, describe duration/location/etc. _____
6. Dressing dry/intact   Yes _____ No _____
   If drainage present, describe _____
7. Is the patient experiencing any of the following?                    Comments
   1. Increased vaginal bleeding        Yes ___ No ___ NA ___   _____
   2. Muscular discomfort               Yes ___ No ___ NA ___   _____
   3. Pain at IV site                   Yes ___ No ___ NA ___   _____
   4. Sore throat/hoarseness            Yes ___ No ___ NA ___   _____
   5. Elevated temp (if yes, _____ F)   Yes ___ No ___ NA ___   _____
   6. Difficulty voiding                Yes ___ No ___ NA ___   _____
   7. Numbness/pain in extremities      Yes ___ No ___ NA ___   _____
   8. Abdominal cramps                  Yes ___ No ___ NA ___   _____
   9. Other problems specific to procedure: _____
      Explain _____

   10. Do you have any bruises, skin abrasions, or other marks on your skin that you did not have before surgery?
       Yes _____ No _____
   11. Were you kept warm enough during surgery and in the post-anesthesia care unit?
       Yes _____ No _____
8. Was SDS and OR nursing care satisfactory?  Yes _____ No _____ Explain if No _____

9. Were family members included in your care and discharge instructions and were their expectations met?
   Yes _____ No _____
   Explain if No _____
10. Were your post-operative instructions clear and relevant to your needs once you returned home?
    Yes _____ No _____
    Explain if No _____
11. Did you experience any "surprises" once home that you were unsure about that had not been addressed?
    Yes _____ No _____ Explain _____

12. What could we do to improve our Outpatient services/care and/or Operating Room care? _____

13. Referral needed?   Yes _____ No _____ If Yes, MD _____ Social Services _____
    Home Health _____ Physical Therapy _____ Other _____
    Referral completed   Date _____ Time _____

**Follow-up Completed By:** _____

**Figure 13–1.** Postprocedure Instruction Sheet
*Source:* Saint Francis Hospital, Memphis, TN.

x-rays, or complex, such as digital subtraction angiography. It would be impossible to review every ambulatory radiologic procedure, but a few are described below. Note that this area overlaps with other specialty procedures, such as cardiology or gastroenterology.

## Diagnostic procedures

Radiologic diagnostic procedures can involve older techniques such as x-rays, or complex techniques such as magnetic resonance imaging (MRI). Results of radiologic exams are usually used to guide the patient's primary physician in caring for that patient. Pediatric patients may require sedation; adult patients may or may not require sedation, depending upon the procedure.

**Computer-assisted scans.** CAT scans, PET scans, and MRI scans yield valuable information in the detection of pathology.

- Common indications: Evaluation of suspected or confirmed disease; visualization of internal structures.

- Complications: CAT and PET scans involve small amounts of radiation; an MRI scan involves no radiation because it is conducted with the use of a super magnet. This magnet can attract any metal prostheses on the patient's body, from aneursym clips in the patient's head to artificial hip joints.

**Arteriograms.** Arteriograms allow physicians to evaluate the condition of peripheral vessels in the body; dye is injected into the vessel and then radiologic films record the status of the vessel. IV access is secured and the patient is often sedated.

- Common indications: Evaluation of suspected or confirmed vascular disease in the peripheral vessels (often vessels in the lower body).

- Complications: Allergic reactions to the dye, hemorrhage, perforation of the artery.

**Contrast studies.** When dyes are injected and films made of the dye's journey in the body or the effect on a part of the body, dynamic contrast studies are being made.

- Common indications: Evaluation of suspected or confirmed disease.

- Complications: Allergic reactions, infection.

## Therapeutic procedures

Therapeutic radiology has become a specialty within the specialty of radiology, due to the rapidly evolving technology in this area.

**Radiation therapy.** Radiation is sometimes used in the treatment of cancer and other pathologic processes.

- Common indications: Destruction of neoplastic lesions and tissue.

- Complications: Malaise, GI upset, nausea and vomiting, anorexia, and other symptoms.

## Nursing considerations for the patient undergoing a radiologic procedure

Below are listed common basic nursing strategies for the ambulatory radiologic patient and the rationale behind each. This is by no means an exhaustive list; detailed information about nursing care can be found in a surgical nursing textbook and other resources.

- Protect yourself with lead shields in areas where you may be exposed to radiation, because radiation is harmful. The minute doses to which the patient is exposed are generally insignificant, but nurses working in these areas are subject to daily exposure. Note that radiation affects more than just the gonads, so nurses not anticipating pregnancy should still shield themselves.

- Guide the patient to an understanding of the nature and purpose of the radiologic procedure, because this helps reduce anxiety. Reassurance and support are often helpful because the radiologist is usually unknown to the patient until time for the procedure, and this may provoke additional anxiety.

- Do not leave patients unnecessarily exposed at any time; this causes most patients distress.

- Follow your institution's policy in preparing patients for MRI, because any metal on or in the patient's body could be affected by the super magnet used in MRI.

- Remember that some patients, while in the MRI scanner, experience claustrophobia and even panic to the extent that the test may have to be aborted. Detection of susceptible patients before the procedure allows an opportunity for the patient to practice relaxation techniques or for the physician to order a tranquilizer before the scan. (This patient will of course then require someone to drive home).

- Note that the nurse involved in administering any sedation or monitoring the patient's condition must have advanced training and skills; see Appendix B, Conscious Sedation.

# CARDIAC PROCEDURES

Cardiac procedures can be relatively minor such as electrocardiograms (ECG) or complex, like arteriograms or angioplasty. Some of these procedures are performed in the cardiologist's office, others in ambulatory units, and still others in the hospital. Some of these procedures also involve radiology or may be performed in the radiology department. As with other specialties, therapeutic procedures are often conducted along with diagnostic procedures if pathology is found.

## Diagnostic procedures

Diagnostic cardiac procedures are generally undertaken to evaluate the structure and/or function of the heart and coronary arteries.

**Echocardiogram.** Using sound waves, this test records the structure of the heart.

- Common indications: Evaluation of suspected heart disease such as valvular deformity; diagnosis of cardiomegaly and pericardial effusions.

- Complications: Rare; echocardiograms are neither stressful nor invasive.

**24-hour (Holter) ECG monitoring.** The patient is connected to a small portable ECG monitor that he or she will wear for at least 24 hours while the heart rhythm is continuously recorded. The patient keeps a diary of activity during this time and makes a notation if any palpitations or chest pain is experienced.

- Common indications: Evaluation of suspected arrhythmias; monitoring of the heart's response to common everyday activities.

- Complications: Rare; possibly skin irritation from electrodes.

**Exercise treadmill test.** While exercising on a treadmill, the patient's heart and vital signs are monitored to evaluate the body's response to the stress of exercise.

- Common indications: Evaluation of suspected ischemic heart disease and chest pain; also performed as a fitness evaluation.

- Complications: Myocardial infarction, cardiovascular collapse can result from this stress test.

**Transesophageal echocardiography (TEE).** This is a variation of the echocardiogram. A tube is placed in the esophagus to generate sound waves; the resulting images are generally of higher quality than the echocardiogram, which examines the heart through the chest wall.

- Common indications: Evaluation of the structures of the heart, including defects in the valves or myocardium.

- Complications: Uncommon, although perforation, hemorrhage, and arrhythmias may develop.

**IV dipyridamole (Persantine) thallium test.** After an IV dose of dipyridamole is injected to dilate the coronary arteries, the radioactive isotope thallium is injected. Special radiology equipment records which arteries have been opened by the dipyridamole and which remain occluded or narrowed in response to the dipyridamole.

- Common indications: Evaluation of suspected coronary artery disease.

- Complications: Arrhythmias, allergic reactions, myocardial infarction.

**Cardiac catheterization.** This is a complex diagnostic procedure used in extensive evaluation of the heart's structure and function. It is usually combined with radiologic recording of the heart (angiography).

- Common indications: Evaluation of heart disease including malformations, shunts, and the coronary arteries.

**Complications:** Arrhythmias, allergic reactions, myocardial infarction, rupture or perforation of the heart, stroke, tamponade, death.

## Therapeutic procedures

Therapeutic cardiac procedures are generally undertaken to treat abnormalities in the structure and/or function of the heart and coronary arteries.

**Angioplasty.** A procedure to widen narrowed arteries without surgery, angioplasty also involves the use of radiography. A balloon-tipped catheter is guided into the affected artery and inflated to compress plaque or obstruction against the walls of the artery; clot-dissolving drugs may also be injected. Lasers or mechanical equipment may be used to physically cut away the obstructing tissue. Urokinase is one of the drugs commonly used to declot an obstructed artery.

- Common indications: Occluded or narrowed artery or arteries.

- Complications: Perforation or rupture of the artery, allergic reactions, arrhythmias, stroke, thrombus formation, myocardial infarction.

**Cardioversion.** Some arrhythmias can be terminated and the heart restored to normal sinus rhythm by defibrillation or countershock; this is cardioversion. The patient receives sedatives or hypnotic agents before the shock is delivered and must be monitored closely after the cardioversion.

- Common indications: Atrial arrhythmias such as atrial flutter that are unresponsive to medication and cause unpleasant symptoms to the patient.

- Complications: Lethal arrhythmias, aspiration.

## Nursing considerations for the patient undergoing a cardiac procedure

Below are listed common basic nursing strategies for the ambulatory cardiac patient and the rationale behind each.

- Use the opportunity of the patient's admission to teach good health habits such as diet, exercise, and smoking cessation; explain the beneficial effects of such habits on the cardiovascular system. As health advocates, nurses would be remiss to let the cardiac patient leave their care without discussing non-pharmacologic and non-surgical factors that reduce or limit heart disease.

- Avoid describing cardioversion as a "shock" to these patients (Lippincott, 1986), because this often causes anticipatory anxiety. Refer to the procedure as cardioversion.

- Monitor cardiology patients closely after invasive procedures, because complications can be swift and serious.

- Explain to the patient what to expect during the procedure, including noises and sensation they might feel or hear. This helps to relieve anxiety.

- Accept the cardiac patient and support person's concerns and let them express their fear and anxiety. These procedures are routine to you but not to the patient. Many laypeople presume any cardiac procedure to be serious or fraught with danger and risk of death.

- Avoid exposing female patients unnecessarily during cardiac procedures; this can embarrass and distress the patient.

- Have oxygen, suction, endotracheal tubes, emergency drugs, manual ventilating bag (Ambu bag) and other emergency equipment immediately available whenever you assist in an invasive cardiac procedure.

# OBSTETRICAL PROCEDURES

A number of tests are performed in the prenatal period to determine fetal well-being. These tests are not without risk however, and there are two patients (mother and child) to manage, not one. Prenatal testing often provokes anxiety in the expectant parents who fear receiving news that all is not well and the painful decisions that may follow. The nurse caring for the pregnant ambulatory patient must therefore function as a support person. Many of these tests are performed in special areas such as obstetrics units, so the personnel are quite familiar with the procedures. Common procedures are reviewed below to enhance your understanding and knowledge of ambulatory procedures for the obstetric patient. These procedures are grouped in invasive and non-invasive categories, since all are diagnostic.

## Invasive procedures

In the pregnant patient, invasive procedures are often performed to determine fetal well-being. Invasive procedures usually involve securing tissues or fluid samples for further evaluation.

**Amniocentesis.** With the patient supine, the physician inserts a needle through the abdomen and into the uterine cavity. Needle placement is often guided by ultrasound; amniotic fluid is withdrawn for analysis. Information gleaned includes presence of many congenital and genetic malformations (such as Down's Syndrome) and fetal maturity. Results of the amniocentesis are often not available for several weeks; this test is usually performed in the second trimester.

**Chorionic Villus Sampling (CVS).** Using a vaginal approach, the physician will insert a needle or catheter into the placenta to retrieve samples for study. Results are generally available in a few days; this test is usually performed in the first trimester.

- Common potential complications: Anytime the uterine cavity is invaded, the potential for infection or fetal harm is present. Invasive procedures also can include the risk of hemorrhage and loss of the pregnancy, although both are uncommon.

## Non-invasive procedures

Fetal well-being is also evaluated during the pregnancy with several tests.

**Oxytocin Challenge Test.** This test involves IV administration of oxytocin to determine how well the fetus can withstand contractions.

**Nonstress test.** The fetal heart rate increases with fetal movement; this test assesses that reaction.

**Ultrasound or sonogram.** Many pregnant women are evaluated at least once during their pregnancy with this test that involves bouncing sound waves off the fetal body to form a computerized image of the fetus.

- Common potential complications: Any test of fetal well-being has the potential to challenge the fetus beyond its ability to respond, and fetal well-being may be compromised.

## Nursing strategies for the obstetric patient

Below are listed common basic nursing strategies for the ambulatory obstetric patient and the rationale behind each.

- Offer support and a nonjudgmental ear to the obstetric patient undergoing prenatal testing. Your patient will often be quite anxious about the possible results of the tests; your supportive presence can help comfort her and may reduce her anxiety.

- Explain the procedure before you begin preparing the patient, so she will know what to expect. This can reduce anxiety.

- Maintain aseptic technique as required during invasive procedures; this helps reduce the potential for infection.

- Note that some patients decline prenatal testing because they will not consider aborting the pregnancy if the results are not favorable. In any case, the patient deserves nonjudgmental support from the nurse.

- Give the patient written instructions as necessary to take home with her so she won't forget essential information you may have already discussed with her.

- Advise the patient to call her doctor if she experiences bleeding, pain, fever, or fluid leaking from the vagina. These could be warning signs of a complication and early intervention can prove to be lifesaving.

- Include the baby's father in the process when possible and if desired by the patient; this can enhance the potential for bonding and reduce stress for both parents.

- Be aware that genetics testing is often a time filled with anxiety and even anticipatory grief for the patient; be supportive and allow your patient to express her feelings.

# PARENTERAL THERAPY

While certain parenteral therapies such as chemotherapy and antibiotic infusions have been performed on an ambulatory basis for a decade or more, some therapies previously performed in the hospital or performed by the physician in his or her office are now moving to ambulatory units. A number of parenteral therapies have also advanced out of the professional setting and now are being performed in the patient's home. Nurses performing these treatments should understand the pharmacology and effects of the drugs and substances they administer; the following serves only as a brief overview.

## Chemotherapy

Administration of drugs to fight cancer is called chemotherapy. The goal of most chemotherapy is to disrupt the ability of cancer cells to reproduce and grow while having minimal effect on healthy tissue. Chemotherapy may be used in connection with surgery and radiation therapy or it may be the sole weapon against cancer. See Table 13-1 for Precautions in Handling Cytotoxic Anticancer Drugs. Chemotherapy is not usually a one-time treatment, it usually involves a number of treatments, as does radiation therapy. The following only serves as a superficial look at chemotherapy in the ambulatory setting; nurses administering chemotherapy should refer to a nursing text about chemotherapy because this is a complex and demanding field.

- Injection: Chemotherapy agents may be infused into a vein; in some cases chemotherapy is injected into an artery or into an isolated area of the body (perfusion and infusion). In some cases, prostate cancer is treated with a synthetic form of luteinizing hormone-releasing hormone known as goserelin acetate implant (Zoladex); this is a capsule that is injected under the skin and slowly releases the hormone over the next 28 days. (Roger, Rosas, O'Hanlon-Nichols, 1994.

- Instillation: Chemotherapy agents may be instilled in a body cavity, as is done in bladder cancer.

- Common potential complications: Chemotherapy is notorious for causing nausea and vomiting (N & V). Other complications can include alopecia, stomatitis, malaise, bone marrow depression, GI disorders, central nervous system changes, and toxicity.

### Nursing strategies for the chemotherapy patient

Below are listed common basic nursing strategies for the ambulatory chemotherapy patient and the rationale behind each.

- Remember that goserelin acetate implant (Zoladex) is a synthetic form of luteinizing hormone-releasing hormone and is not a chemotherapeutic agent. Even though prescribed in treatment of bladder cancer, you need wear only gloves during the procedure, as you would do when handling sharps (Roger, Rosas, & O'Hanlon-Nichols, 1994.

- Note that a relatively new drug, ondansetron (Zofran) shows promise in reducing N & V associated with chemotherapy. Propofol (Diprivan) is a hypnotic (see Chapter 5, General Anesthesia) with antiemetic properties that is showing promise in reducing or preventing nausea during chemotherapy (Shafer, 1993).

- Teach the patient and support person about the chemotherapy and what to expect. Make certain they know the name of the chemotherapeutic drug the patient is receiving, because this information can be important to other health care providers who care for the patient. For example, bleomycin (Blenoxane) can lead to pulmonary dysfunction; doxorubicin (Adriamycin) can be cardiotoxic.

- Follow your institution's policy when handling chemotherapeutic agents because these are potentially toxic substances.

- Monitor the intravenous infusion of chemotherapeutic agents because infiltration or extravasation into surrounding tissue can lead to tissue necrosis.

- Advise the patient to avoid contact with people who are or may be ill. Immunosuppression often develops with chemotherapy and the patient may be especially vulnerable to viruses and bacteria.

---

**Table 13-1
Nursing Precautions in Handling Cytotoxic Anticancer Drugs**

**For Personal Safety to Protect Skin and Eyes:**

- Wash hands before and after admixing.
- Wear long-sleeved gown and disposable polyvinyl gloves.
- Wear a mask and safety glasses in absence of a vertical flow hood.
- Hold drug ampules away from the face when they are being opened to remove contents. Cover ampule completely with a gauze pad prior to breaking.
- Wash contaminated skin and surfaces with copious amounts of soap and water.

*Source:* Lippincott Manual of Nursing Practice, 4th ed. 1986.

---

**Antibiotics.** Patients requiring prolonged antibiotic therapy (as in Lyme Disease) often are treated at home, but some may come to the hospital's ambulatory unit for administration of these drugs. The nurse must be certain that the drug is administered correctly without extravasation or infiltration. Sometimes the patient has an indwelling central catheter in place; you should be trained in administration of drugs through this route before you begin an infusion.

**Blood and blood products.** Ambulatory units have been infusing blood and blood products for over a decade, indeed some of these transfusions are now being performed in the patient's home. However, transfusions are still a duty of many ambulatory patient care nurses.

### Nursing strategies for the patient receiving blood products

Below are listed common basic nursing strategies for the ambulatory patient receiving blood products by transfusion.

- Follow facility policy in verifying that you are administering the right product to the right patient; have another professional check also. Administering blood products to the wrong patient can result in patient death.

- Stay with the patient during the initial infusion; this enables you to assess the patient for a reaction which is most likely to occur soon after beginning the infusion.

- Use filters and warming units only when approved by the blood bank supplying the product or your facility. Warming blood in the sink or microwave is inappropriate and dangerous.

# OTHER AMBULATORY PROCEDURES

There is an ever increasing variety of procedures now moving into the ambulatory care field. Below are briefly addressed some of the other patients and procedures an ambulatory patient care nurse might encounter:

- Hydration: Patients who are dehydrated from vomiting or other illness sometimes come to the ambulatory unit for hydration with IV fluids.

- Dialysis: Renal dialysis patients are sometimes seen in ambulatory surgery units when they come for shunt placement or revisions, or for thrombolysis and angioplasty of a blocked dialysis graft. Dialysis is of course commonly performed on an ambulatory basis, and specialized freestanding units exist all across the country for just this purpose.

- Electroconvulsive therapy (ECT): ECT is the application of an electric shock to the brain; a convulsion follows but the neuromuscular effects are minimized by the prior administration of a neuromuscular blocking drug such as succinylcholine. While this technique has fallen in and out favor, it is still performed on psychiatric patients, mostly those suffering from severe depression. ECT is often performed in the postanesthesia care unit and the patient receives a hypnotic agent along with the neuromuscular blocking agent. Respirations must be supported; aspiration is possible.

- Bone marrow aspiration and biopsy: Bone marrow may be aspirated from the iliac crest or sternum in an effort to establish a diagnosis or to monitor the progression of pathology. These patients may receive sedation and so must be monitored carefully by the nurse and must be driven home by their support person.

# PAIN MANAGEMENT

Specialized clinics have opened in the past decade solely for the purpose of treating patients with chronic pain; some hospitals use the postanesthesia care unit or ambulatory unit to administer pain control treatments. Usually staffed by anesthesiologists, these clinics may also employ a multidisciplinary team approach to treating chronic pain.

### Nerve blocks

Specific nerves may be blocked with local anesthetics injected concurrently with a steroid to reduce inflammation in the painful area. Sometimes a toxic agent is injected to destroy the nerve in hopes of relieving the pain.

- Stellate ganglion: In the treatment of herpes zoster, stellate ganglion blocks can relieve pain (Currey & Dalsania, 1991). Accidental intravascular injection can cause a seizure and cardiovascular collapse; airway compromise is unusual but possible.

- Epidural: Steroids and local anesthetics may be injected in the epidural space in an effort at relieving chronic neck and back pain. Complications can include inadvertent systemic injection of the LA with resulting seizures and cardiovascular collapse; a hematoma may form at the injection site and compress vital nerves, thereby necessitating emergency surgery.

- Intercostal block: Local anesthetics may be injected in the intercostal spaces (between the ribs) in order to temporarily relieve pain in the chest, such as from breast cancer. Puncture of the lung and pneumothorax are potential complications.

**Other therapies.** Devices may be applied externally or implanted in the ambulatory patient in an effort at managing pain. Complications during and after these pain therapies depend on the procedure and the patient.

# PULMONARY PROCEDURES

A number of pulmonary procedures are performed on ambulatory patients, including both diagnostic testing and therapeutic procedures performed in surgery.

**Bronchoscopy.** This procedure may be done under general anesthesia in the operating room, or with local anesthesia in a special procedure room or with conscious sedation. The purpose is to visualize the airways and secure specimens that will aid in diagnosis and treatment of the patient. Bronchoscopy may also be used therapeutically.

**Pulmonary function studies.** This is a series of tests to evaluate the function and capabilities of the pulmonary system. This may be performed on an ambulatory basis in a patient scheduled for major surgery, or in a patient with pulmonary complaints.

- Complications: As with any procedure, complications can be minor or severe. Because pulmonary procedures involve manipulation of the airways, hypoxia and airway compromise are possible. Nurses involved in administering sedation or monitoring the patient must have advanced skills and training.

# SUMMARY

This chapter reviewed common diagnostic and therapeutic ambulatory procedures in the following classifications: gastroenterology, radiology, cardiology, obstetrics, parenteral therapy, pulmonary, pain management, and others. Common complications and nursing strategies associated with each were reviewed. Since it would be impossible to discuss or review every ambulatory diagnostic or therapeutic procedure here, this chapter served as an overview and introduction.

# CRITICAL CONCEPTS

- You should take personal and environmental safety measures whenever you administer chemotherapy or are exposed to radiation.

- Changes in health care mean that nurses are being asked to perform procedures that in the past would have been performed in the physician's office or hospital.

- Always check and double-check when administering medications, and be aware that administration of a blood product or toxic chemotherapy agent to the wrong patient could cause the patient's death.

- Patients are often quite concerned about undergoing diagnostic tests; this concern seems heightened in cardiac and obstetric patients, so they often require extra reassurance and more explanations than usual.

# EXAM QUESTIONS

## Chapter 13

Questions 86-92

86. Notify the radiology staff if your patient has any metal protheses (such as artificial joints or surgical clips) and is undergoing a(n):

    a. CAT scan
    b. PET scan
    c. MRI scan
    d. OBS scan

87. A procedure to clear narrowed arteries without surgery is:

    a. cardiac catheterization
    b. angioplasty
    c. ileostomy
    d. arthroplasty

88. A common nursing diagnosis for cardiac and obstetric patients is:

    a. injury
    b. fear
    c. verbal communication impairment
    d. incontinence

89. Your pregnant patient had an amniocentesis one hour ago. As you assist her to stand and dress, a large volume of fluid gushes from her vagina. You should:

    a. find her a clean gown to wear home
    b. notify the physician immediately
    c. reassure her and help her into her car
    d. advise her to call her doctor if it happens again

90. Injection of goserelin acetate implant (Zoladex) is:

    a. subcutaneous
    b. intramuscular
    c. intravenous
    d. intrathecal

91. Which of the following structures is subject to perforation during esophagogastroduodenoscopy (EGD)?

    a. esophagus
    b. biliary tract
    c. ileocecal valve
    d. colon

92. Goserelin acetate implant (Zoladex) is used in the treatment of:

    a. prostate cancer
    b. liver disease
    c. breast cancer
    d. skin cancer

# CHAPTER 14

# SURGICAL AND ANESTHETIC EMERGENCIES

## CHAPTER OBJECTIVE

After completing this chapter, you should be better prepared to anticipate, identify, and intervene in surgical and anesthetic emergencies.

## LEARNING OBJECTIVES

After reading this chapter, you should be able to:

1. Select potential nursing diagnoses for ambulatory patients experiencing an anesthetic or surgical emergency.

2. Identify serious and grave anesthetic and surgical emergencies.

3. Specify nursing measures that enhance the potential for a favorable outcome from the untoward event.

4. Recognize symptoms and treatment of malignant hyperthermia.

5. Specify common interventions in cardiovascular and airway emergencies.

## INTRODUCTION

Most ambulatory patients come and go with their care uninterrupted by complications. Untoward events, if any, generally revolve around concerns such as nausea and vomiting or pain management; these were discussed in earlier chapters. However, as stressed in earlier chapters, just because a procedure can be performed on an ambulatory basis does not mean that it is minor or risk-free. This is especially true of ambulatory surgical procedures. This chapter reviews serious or potentially fatal emergencies that, while rare, may arise during the perioperative period. Emergencies associated with surgery are reviewed first; complications associated with anesthesia follow. Because patients don't have anesthesia without surgery (except in pain management and labor), you will note that these two fields intertwine and many surgical and anesthetic complications are linked. The nurse is an essential member of the team facing surgical and anesthetic emergencies. In fact, the nurse's actions may be the pivotal point in determining the outcome. The information in this chapter is presented to enhance your knowledge of critical events so that you can be better prepared in the event you face one of the challenges, and so you will have more confidence in addressing your patient's concerns. A summary and a review of the critical concepts presented close the chapter. Complications that may develop during special ambulatory procedures are discussed in Chapter 13.

# SURGICAL EMERGENCIES

Most surgical procedures are completed in a routine manner without incident. However, surgical emergencies can result in serious complications or even patient death. Surgical complications that occur in the perioperative period may involve technical errors and volume depletion.

**Technical errors.** Technical errors in surgery range from untoward accidents related to surgical technique, to operating on the wrong part of the body. Examples would be puncturing the bowel during laparoscopy or operating on the wrong knee during arthroscopy. Other surgical complications can arise when pathology is more advanced than anticipated. This usually results in more extensive surgery than might have been originally planned and the patient may need to be admitted to a hospital for postoperative care.

**Volume depletion.** Volume depletion in surgery can result from excessive blood loss or inadequate fluid replacement during the procedure. Patients whose condition was less than optimal before the procedure, such as those with a low hematocrit, are especially vulnerable. After completion of surgery, postoperative bleeding may necessitate a return to surgery to halt the blood loss. Postoperative bleeding may be occult and heralded only by the signs of volume depletion such as hypotension, tachycardia, and oliguria. Postoperative bleeding may also be overt, with a hematoma forming at the incision site.

Nursing care in these surgical emergencies revolves around assessing the patient, securing supplies such as intravenous (IV) fluids or blood products for infusion, assisting the team as necessary, and informing the family as indicated by the surgeon. Table 14-1 lists common potential nursing diagnoses for patients experiencing a surgical complication.

# ANESTHETIC EMERGENCIES

Advances in pharmacology and technology make anesthesia safer than ever, and most patients do quite well. But the nature of the human body means that emergencies can develop at any time. The most serious complications that develop during anesthesia are associated with airway compromise, cardiac compromise, and a hypermetabolic crisis known as malignant hyperthermia. These are discussed below.

## Airway compromise

As all nurses know, maintaining a patent airway is always the first priority in any patient: no airway, no patient. Airway compromise is always an emergency, since death can follow in a matter of minutes if the airway is not restored. Three different types of airway compromise you may see in the perioperative period include: laryngospasm, difficult intubation, and pulmonary aspiration.

- Laryngospasm: Sudden spasmodic closure of the vocal cords is called laryngospasm; this closure will occlude the flow of air into the trachea and the lungs. If you've ever swallowed food or liquid and had it "go down the wrong way" then subsequently coughed and choked, you've had a laryngospasm. In most cases, this resolves spontaneously, although there are some tense moments when the patient exhibits inspiratory stridor, or makes a crowing sound as he or she tries to inhale. However, laryngospasm may persist and the patient can become hypoxic. Untreated, death can result. Treatment consists of removing the irritating stimulus, which may be

### Table 14-1
### Potential Nursing Diagnoses for Ambulatory Patients Experiencing Surgical Emergencies

| Nursing Diagnosis | Nursing intervention |
|---|---|
| Cardiac output, decreased due to reduced stroke volume related to hemorrhage | Know in advance which patients will refuse blood transfusions; inform other team members. In the event of significant surgical blood loss, assist surgical team by securing supplies and instruments needed to obtain hemostasis; assist anesthetist fluid replacement by retrieving and checking blood products and other intravenous fluids for infusion. Consult with surgeon regarding notification of patient's support person or family of this complication. Know the location of the emergency code cart and have it ready in the event of cardiovascular collapse. |
| Fluid volume deficit from active loss | Measure and record urine output; assist surgical team in hemostasis and anesthetist in fluid replacement as necessary. |
| Tissue perfusion alteration related to decreased arterial blood flow and hypovolemia | Monitor and record amount of blood loss during surgery; administer emergency drugs as ordered and in accordance with facility policy; assist with positioning patient to maximize blood flow and tissue perfusion; secure emergency drugs and equipment in the event it is needed. |
| Grieving, anticipatory related to potential loss of patient (Family or support person) | Inform support person and/or family of surgical emergency or complication as allowed by physician in charge. Help support person to identify people such as relatives or clergy whose presence could be comforting during crisis; notify those people (with the support person's permission). Stay with support person, do not offer false reassurances, allow person to express feelings and concerns. |

Please note this is a sample of potential nursing diagnoses and is not presented as, nor intended to be, a complete care plan for the ambulatory patient. More complete information can be found in a medical surgical nursing course and textbook.

Adapted from: *Nursing Diagnosis Reference Manual* by Sheila Sparks and Cynthia M. Taylor, Springhouse Corporation, 1991, and *Overview of Anesthesia* for Nurses by L. Chitwood, Western Schools, 1992.

an oral airway or secretions, and positive pressure ventilation by mask with oxygen to force air past the cords. In some cases the laryngospasm persists and no air can be forced past the cords, so administration of a short-acting muscle relaxant may be necessary to break the spasm. In this case, the patient must be artificially ventilated until respirations resume.

- Difficult intubation: During anesthesia, the anesthetist maintains the patency of the patient's airway. In most cases this is a routine task that is accomplished by positioning of the head and mandible, and/or by the use of artificial devices such as oral airways, nasal airways, and endotracheal tubes. Endotracheal tubes are used during most general anesthetics other than very brief procedures such as a D & C, or whenever the patient is at risk for aspiration. Sometimes insertion of the endotracheal tube into the trachea is difficult or impossible; this is referred to as a difficult intubation. Inability to place an endotracheal tube or maintain the patient's airway can lead to hypoxia and patient death. In many cases, patients who may be difficult to intubate can be detected before surgery. These are patients who are obese, have short thick necks, receding mandibles, or limited range of motion of the head, neck, or temporomandibular joint. But difficult intubation can also be totally unexpected in certain patients. Whatever the cause, the patient should be ventilated by mask; if this is impossible then another method of delivering oxygen to the lungs must be established. This may include a tracheotomy or cricothyroidotomy, where a large bore intravenous catheter is inserted into the trachea and connected to an oxygen source. Appendix C is an algorithm for management of difficult airway.

- Aspiration: During general anesthesia, protective airway reflexes are suppressed. Because of this, anything in the patient's stomach could reflux back up into the throat and be inhaled into the patient's lungs. This is called aspiration. It only takes a small amount of aspirated gastric secretions (25 cc) to damage the lungs; this can result in a fatal pneumonia. Prevention is easier than treatment. In some ambulatory units, patients are routinely medicated with an aspiration prophylaxis protocol that may include a histamine blocker such as ranitidine (Zantac) to raise the pH of the stomach contents, a GI stimulant such as metoclopramide (Reglan) to hasten emptying of the stomach, and a clear, non-particulate antacid such as sodium citrate (Bicitra) to neutralize remaining secretions. Opinions on the value of this prophylaxis are constantly changing; you should monitor this field for developments. Patients especially at risk for aspiration include those with hiatal hernia, pregnant or obese patients, and those who have not been NPO. In this case, the anesthetist may ask the nurse to apply pressure to the cricoid cartilage in the patient's neck during induction of anesthesia. This maneuver helps seal off the esophagus and stomach contents from the trachea. This pressure should not be released until the cuff on the endotracheal tube is inflated to accomplish the same purpose, or until the anesthetist asks you to release it. Should aspiration occur, cardiac arrest and hypoxia may result. Treatment is supportive and symptomatic.

## Cardiovascular compromise

Cardiovascular compromise can develop as a result of surgery or anesthesia and must be evaluated promptly. Common cardiovascular crises during surgery include arrhythmias and volume imbalance.

- Arrhythmias: Modern anesthetic agents are much safer than obsolete agents such as ether, so cardiac arrhythmias don't develop as often. Nevertheless, arrhythmias can develop during anesthesia and surgery. The local anesthetic (LA) cocaine or other LAs containing epinephrine can trigger cardiac arrhythmias, especially when used with older inhalation agents such as halothane. Arrhythmias may also be the result of catecholamine (stress hormones) release or surgical stimulation, as in a vagal response. In healthy patients, many arrhythmias are generally benign and require no treatment. When necessary, treatment involves removing the stimulus (such as deepening anesthesia or avoiding cocaine and epinephrine use) and administration of cardiac agents as indicated to control the arrhythmia. Sudden cardiac arrest is rare during surgery; there are generally prodromal signs.

- Volume imbalance: Excessive blood loss and/or inadequate fluid replacement contribute to cardiovascular instability. Anesthetic agents also depress the cardiovascular system to some degree; this can result in hypotension and decreased perfusion. As noted in Chapter 5, the anesthetist must strike a balance between adequate anesthesia so the surgeon can operate, and maintenance of the patient's cardiorespiratory system.

## Malignant hyperthermia

In susceptible patients, exposure to certain anesthetic agents results in a fulminant hypermetabolic crisis called Malignant Hyperthermia (MH). Marked by increased body temperature, tachycardia, rigidity of the muscles, and cardiac arrhythmias, MH can cause cardiovascular collapse and death. A genetic disorder that triggers an abnormal response to anesthetic agents, MH is rare. Unfortunately, when MH occurs it is a life threatening emergency. MH is frequently fatal within minutes, so early recognition and treatment is crucial. Older children and young adults are most frequently affected; males more often than females (Donnelly, 1994). Ideally, MH susceptible patients are identified before administration of anesthesia; patients are questioned about unusual responses blood relatives may have had to anesthesia. MH can also develop during the postoperative period, or recur after an initial episode is successfully treated. Treatment involves halting the anesthetic and surgery, administering dantrolene (Dantrium), cooling the patient by any means possible, and supporting the vital functions.

Table 14-2 lists potential nursing diagnoses for the ambulatory patient experiencing an anesthetic complication.

# NURSING STRATEGIES

Nursing intervention in grave or life threatening emergencies requires skill and knowledge; detailed information can be found in nursing textbooks. Below however, are basic nursing strategies and the rationale behind each. As always, your intervention should be within the scope of your institution's practice guidelines, consistent your state's Nurse Practice Act and your license, and commensurate with your skills and training.

- Know in advance of need where emergency supplies are kept and how to call for emergency teams. Know where dantrolene (Dantrium) and iced IV solutions are kept. In the event of a patient crisis, seconds count and time spent looking up a number or searching for supplies lessens the probability of a good outcome.

- Verify with the patient, not just the chart, on which part of the body surgery is to be performed. This reduces the chance of error that could have disastrous consequences.

- Stay near to the patient's support person or family during a time of crisis and give them reports on the patient's condition as allowed by the physician in charge. Certain information is best given by the surgeon or anesthetist involved, but your presence can be reassuring and supportive.

- Offer to call friends, clergy, social workers or counselors to assist in supporting the family member or support person during a serious complication. Under stress, neither the patient nor the support person may think of this, but the presence of crisis professionals or close friends may be helpful during this time.

- Provide the support person or family with a private place to wait during or after a serious complication. This can be a difficult time and they are entitled to privacy; secluding the family also results in less alarm to other patients and families.

- Follow your facility's policy in documenting complications. Some facilities have special reports that must be sent to the facility's risk management department but are not part of the patient's record.

- Maintain certification in Basic Life Support and consider studying for certification in Advanced Cardiac Life Support. The skills and knowledge

## Table 14-2
## Potential Nursing Diagnoses for Ambulatory Patients Experiencing Anesthetic Emergencies

### DIFFICULT INTUBATION

| Nursing Diagnosis | Nursing Intervention |
|---|---|
| Gas exchange impairment related to altered oxygen supply; (inability to deliver oxygen to the lungs) | Know the location of the emergency tracheotomy tray. |
| Airway clearance, ineffective related to tracheobronchial obstruction | Note that surgery should not begin until the patient's airway is secured. |
| Suffocation, potential | Assist the anesthesia team as necessary with suctioning, passing or securing supplies, and applying cricoid pressure. |

### ASPIRATION

| Nursing Diagnosis | Nursing Intervention |
|---|---|
| Gas exchange impairment related to altered oxygen-carrying capacity of the blood (due to aspiration) | Know the location of emergency drugs, defibrillator, tracheotomy tray. |
| Aspiration related to absence of protective mechanisms | Assist the anesthesia team as necessary with suctioning, passing or securing supplies and medications, and applying cricoid pressure if requested. |
| Suffocation, potential | Do not release cricoid pressure on the neck until the anesthetist asks you to, if you are assisting with intubation. Releasing pressure before the endotracheal tube is correctly placed and the cuff is inflated can result in aspiration. |

# Table 14-2 (cont.)
## Potential Nursing Diagnoses for Ambulatory Patients Experiencing Anesthetic Emergencies

### MALIGNANT HYPERTHERMIA

| Nursing Diagnosis | Nursing Intervention |
|---|---|
| Thermoregulation, ineffective, related to illness (MH)<br><br>Gas exchange impairment related to altered oxygen-carrying capacity of the blood<br><br>Tissue perfusion alteration, arterial and venous | Know the location of MH treatment supplies and obtain them as ordered.<br><br>Assist the anesthesia team as necessary with cooling the patient, securing emergency drugs as needed, passing supplies.<br><br>Keep family informed as necessary; consult with the anesthesia team and surgeon about this. |

### CARDIAC ARREST, HYPOTENSION, ARRHYTHMIAS

| Nursing Diagnosis | Nursing Intervention |
|---|---|
| Tissue perfusion alteration related to reduced venous and/or arterial blood flow<br><br>Cardiac output, decreased, related to reduced stroke volume as a result of electrophysiologic problems | Know the location of emergency drugs and defibrillator.<br><br>Assist the anesthesia team as necessary with passing or securing supplies and medications; hang blood as ordered after following institutional guidelines for blood transfusion.<br><br>Note time of events and document record according to institutional guidelines. |

*Please note this is a sample of potential nursing diagnoses and interventions; and is not presented as, nor intended to be, a complete plan of care for these anesthetic emergencies. More complete information can be found in a medical surgical nursing text or anesthesia reference text.*

*Source: Overview of Anesthesia for Nurses by L. Chitwood, Western Schools, 1992, and adapted from Nursing Diagnosis Reference Manual by Sheila Sparks and Cynthia M. Taylor, Springhouse Corporation, 1991.*

gleaned from these courses will increase your confidence and enable you to react efficiently in a crisis.

- Recommend that the patient's support person or family remain in the facility while the patient is in surgery. While complications and emergencies are rare, life threatening crises can and do develop. Such an occurrence is tragic enough without having to wait until the patient's support person or family returns late in the afternoon to pick up the patient only then to be told that the patient died that morning or has been transferred to a critical care facility.

- Know before surgery which patients refuse administration of blood products, document that decision according to facility policy, and inform the other members of the perioperative team of the patient's decision. An increasing number of patients are reluctant to sign a consent authorizing blood transfusion due to fear of transmittable diseases such as hepatitis or AIDS; many Jehovah's Witnesses routinely refuse transfusion. Most ambulatory surgery procedures involve little potential for significant blood loss, but complications are always possible. Knowing in advance can help direct you and the team to alternatives, such as autologous blood donations. In this situation, the patient donates his or her own blood which is collected and stored until surgery, when it can be reinfused as needed.

- Follow institutional policy when administering blood to a patient. This usually includes a protocol for the infusion and patient identification. Following the policy will help reduce the potential for errors with serious consequences.

- Note the time when critical events occur and document these for the record. In an emergency, one person is often designated just to record times and document responses on the record. Accuracy will be helpful in follow-up care of the patient and may prove crucial in the event of litigation.

- Call for all available help immediately in an MH crisis, because extra people will be needed to assist in the crisis and retrieve supplies. Assist in cooling the patient by any means possible during an MH crisis. Secure iced IV fluids, and prepare to lavage body cavities such as the colon, stomach, and bladder with chilled solutions in an attempt to reduce the patient's temperature. Secure large quantities of ice in the event the team elects to pack the patient in ice. Know the location of dantrolene (Dantrium) and how to mix it for use by the anesthesia team. Note that the anesthesia machine in use at the time of the MH crisis is usually immediately exchanged for another machine, in case some of the triggering agent still remains in the first machine.

- Learn how to properly apply cricoid pressure. This skill is vital whenever a patient at risk for reflux is intubated, this includes patients who require emergency intubation. Improper application can damage the trachea and be ineffective in preventing aspiration. Once you are properly applying pressure as requested by the anesthetist, do not release it until you are told to do so because this could result in aspiration.

- Do not offer nourishment to the postop patient until you feel certain the potential for postoperative complications are past, because if the patient did have to return to surgery the risk of aspiration would be increased.

# SUMMARY

This chapter reviewed serious or potentially fatal emergencies that, while rare, may arise during the perioperative period. Emergencies associated with

# CHAPTER 14 —
## SURGICAL AND ANESTHETIC EMERGENCIES

surgery were reviewed first; emergencies associated with anesthesia followed. It was demonstrated that the nurse is an essential member of the team facing surgical and anesthetic emergencies. In fact, the nurse's actions may be the pivotal point in determining the outcome.

# CRITICAL CONCEPTS

- The perioperative nurse's actions significantly influence the outcome of complications.

- You should not circulate or scrub on a surgical case unless you know the location of the emergency code crash cart, malignant hyperthermia supplies, emergency airway management equipment, and iced IV fluids.

- While rare, surgical and anesthetic complications can be serious or fatal.

- Malignant hyperthermia is a hypermetabolic crisis triggered in susceptible individuals by certain anesthetic agents; it is frequently fatal. Treatment includes administering dantrolene (Dantrium).

# EXAM QUESTIONS

## Chapter 14

Questions 93-100

93. The drug specific to treatment of malignant hyperthermia (MH) is:

    a. metoclopramide (Reglan)
    b. esmolol (Brevibloc)
    c. sodium citrate (Bicitra)
    d. dantrolene (Dantrium)

94. Treatment of MH may include:

    a. packing the patient in ice
    b. applying patient warming devices
    c. performing range of motion exercises
    d. suctioning the oropharnyx

95. During intubation, aspiration may be prevented by application of:

    a. cricoid pressure
    b. positive ventilation
    c. halo tongs
    d. trachea dam

96. A sign of malignant hyperthermia is:

    a. tachycardia
    b. increased intracranial pressure
    C. oliguria
    d. pneumonia

97. Inhalation of the stomach contents into the lungs is called:

    a. enuresis
    b. gastritis
    c. difficult intubation
    d. aspiration

98. When attempts at intubation fail, an emergency method sometimes used to deliver oxygen to the lungs is:

    a. tracheoscopy
    b. cricothyroidotomy
    c. cystoscopy
    d. laminectomy

99. During airway compromise, the nurse may be asked to assist by:

    a. administering wet to dry soaks
    b. placing the patient in trendelenburg position
    c. intubating the patient
    d. applying cricoid pressure

100. Suffocation, potential related to external factors is a nursing diagnosis for the patient experiencing which emergency?

    a. malignant hyperthermia
    b. cardiac arrhythmias
    c. difficult intubation
    d. hypovolemic shock

# APPENDIX A

American Academy of Ambulatory Care Nursing
East Holly Avenue
Box 56
Pitman, NJ 08071-0056

Accreditation Association for Ambulatory Health Care, Inc.
9933 Lawler Ave.
Skokie, IL 60077-3702

American Academy of Ambulatory Nursing Administrators
North Woodbury Rd. Box 56
Pitman, NJ 08071

American Association of Nurse Anesthetists
216 Higgins Rd.
Park Ridge, IL 60068-5790

American Society of Anesthesiologists
520 N. Northwest Hwy
Park Ridge, IL 60068-1573

American Society of Post Anesthesia Nurses
11512 Allecingie Pkwy.
Richmond, VA 23235

Association of Operating Room Nurses
2170 S. Parker #300
Denver, CO 80231-5711

Federated Ambulatory Surgery Association
700 N. Fairfax #520
Alexandria, VA 22314

Malignant Hyperthermia Association
P. O. Box 191
Westport, CT 06881-0191

North American Nursing Diagnosis Association
3525 Caroline St.
St. Louis, MO 63104

# APPENDIX B

## ASSOCIATION OF OPERATING ROOM NURSES RECOMMENDED PRACTICES

## Monitoring the Patient Receiving IV Concious Sedation

## Recommended Practice I

**The nurse should know the goals and objectives of IV conscious sedation.**

*Interpretive statement 1:*

The primary goal of IV conscious sedation is allaying patient fear and anxiety regarding the planned procedure.

*Rationale:*

Adequate preprocedure preparation and verbal reassurance from nursing personnel facilitate the effects of IV conscious sedation and may allow for a decrease in the dosage of opioids, benzodiazepines, and sedatives used.

*Interpretive statement 2:*

Objectives for the patient receiving IV conscious sedation include
- alteration of mood,
- maintenance of consciousness,
- cooperation,
- elevation of pain threshold,
- minimal variation of vital signs,
- some degree of amnesia, and
- a rapid, safe return to ambulation.

*Rationale:*

Intravenous conscious sedation produces a condition where the patient exhibits a depressed level of consciousness but retains the ability to independently and continuously maintain a patent airway and respond appropriately to verbal commands or physical stimulation. Misunderstanding the objectives of IV conscious sedation may jeopardize the quality of care.

## Recommended Practice II

**Each patient receiving IV conscious sedation should be assessed physiologically and psychologically before the procedure.**

*Interpretive statement 1:*

Preprocedure assessment should include
- physical assessment,
- current medications,
- drug allergies/sensitivities,
- concurrent medical problems (eg, hypertension, diabetes, cardiopulmonary disease, kidney problems, respiratory problems),
- history of substance abuse,
- chief complaint,
- baseline vital signs, including height, weight, and age,
- level of consciousness,
- emotional state,
- communication ability, and
- perceptions regarding procedure and sedation.

*Rationale:*

Preprocedure assessment provides baseline data and identifies patient risk factors.

## Recommended Practice III

**Each patient receiving IV conscious sedation should be monitored for reaction to drugs and for physiological and psychological changes.**

*Interpretive statement 1:*

The nurse managing the care of the patient should "have no other responsibilities that would leave the patient unattended or compromise continuous monitoring."

*Rationale:*

Agents administered for IV conscious sedation may cause behavioral changes and rapid, adverse physiological changes. It is unrealistic to assume that one nurse could perform circulating duties and also provide continuous monitoring, physical care, and emotional support for the patient.

*Interpretive statement 2:*

The nurse who is monitoring the patient should be aware of the desirable and undesirable effects of IV conscious sedation.

*Rationale:*

Observation of the patient for desired therapeutic drug effects, prevention of adverse effects, early detection of nonpreventable adverse effects, and accurate documentation of the patient's response are integral components of the monitoring process.

*Discussion:*

Desirable effects of IV conscious sedation include
- intact protective reflexes,
- relaxation,
- cooperation,
- diminished verbal communication, and
- easy arousal from sleep.

Undesirable effects of IV conscious sedation include
- nystagmus (may be normal with large doses of diazepam),
- slurred speech,
- unarousable sleep,
- hypotension,
- agitation,
- combativeness,
- hypoventilation,
- respiratory depression,
- airway obstruction, and
- apnea.

*Interpretive statement 3:*

Before IV sedation is administered, the patient should have oxygen delivery in place, IV access line established, and monitoring in place.

Monitoring parameters should include
- respiratory rate,
- oxygen saturation,
- blood pressure,
- cardiac rate and rhythm,
- level of consciousness, and
- skin condition.

Changes in patient condition should be reported immediately to the physician.

*Rationale:*

Sedatives and benzodiazepines used for IV conscious sedation may cause somnolence, confusion, coma, diminished reflexes, and depressed respiratory and cardiovascular function. Opioids used for IV conscious sedation may cause respiratory depression, hypotension, nausea, and vomiting. Overdosage and adverse reactions may occur any time during the procedure and may be reversible.

*Interpretive statement 4:*

Each patient receiving IV conscious sedation should have continuous IV access.

*Rationale:*

Continuous IV access provides a means for administering drugs used for IV conscious sedation and for implementing corrective measures for adverse effects (ie, drug and fluid administration).

*Discussion:*

Continuous IV access may be obtained by use of a heparin lock device or infusion of IV fluids. Type of access chosen will vary depending on institutional policy and physician preference.

*Interpretive statement 5:*

An emergency cart with appropriate emergency resuscitative drugs and a defibrillator should be immediately available to every location where IV conscious sedation is administered.

*Rationale:*

Overdose or adverse reactions may cause respiratory depression, hypotension, and impaired cardiovascular function requiring resuscitation.

*Interpretive statement 6:*

The following equipment should be present and ready for use in the room where IV conscious sedation is administered:
- oxygen,
- suction,
- bag and mask devices,
- oral, nasopharyngeal airways, and endotracheal tubes in various sizes,
- sphygmomanometer or noninvasive blood pressure monitor,
- electrocardiograph, and
- pulse oximeter.

*Rationale:*

Equipment for resuscitation or drug reversal efforts should be present because diminished reflexes, depressed respiratory function, and impaired cardiovascular function may occur with drugs used for IV conscious sedation.

## Recommended Practice IV

**The nurse monitoring the patient should have a working knowledge of resuscitation equipment and the function and use of monitoring equipment and should be able to interpret the data obtained.**

*Interpretive statement 1:*

The nurse monitoring the patient should know how to operate and troubleshoot monitoring equipment used with the patient receiving IV conscious sedation.

*Rationale:*

Knowledge of the functions and proper use of monitoring equipment is essential for providing safe care.

*Interpretive statement 2:*

The nurse monitoring the patient should be able to demonstrate acquired knowledge of
- anatomy and physiology,
- pharmacology of drugs used for IV conscious sedation,
- cardiac arrhythmia interpretation,
- complications related to the use of IV conscious sedation,
- principles of oxygen delivery, and
- respiratory physiology, transport, and uptake.

*Rationale:*

Drugs used for IV conscious sedation may cause rapid, adverse physiologic responses in the patient. Early detection of such responses allows for rapid intervention and treatment.

*Interpretive statement 3:*

The nurse monitoring the patient should be skilled in the use of oxygen delivery devices and airway management.

*Rationale:*

Rapid intervention is necessary in the event of complications from the undesired effects of the IV conscious sedation.

*Discussion:*

The airway management skill level of the nurse monitoring the patient should be defined by institutional policy. Basic cardiac life support, which includes maintenance of a patent airway by use of the head-tilt/chin-lift maneuver, is considered basic for all nurses. The use of oxygen delivery devices (eg, bag and mask devices) may be included as part of the orientation and continuing education process for nurses who will be monitoring patients receiving IV conscious sedation. Advanced cardiac life support certification may be required by some institutions. Persons with such skills (eg, code team, anesthesia personnel) should be readily available to the location where IV conscious sedation is being administered.

## Recommended Practice V

**Documentation on the patient record during the administration of IV conscious sedation should reflect evidence of continued assessment, diagnosis, outcome identification, planning, implementation, and evaluation of patient care.**

*Interpretive statement 1:*

Documentation should include
- dosage, route, time, and effects of all drugs or agents used,
- type and amount of fluids administered, including blood and blood products, monitoring devices or equipment used,
- physiologic data from continuous monitoring documented at 5- to 15-minute intervals and at any significant event,
- level of consciousness,
- any interventions and the patient's responses, and
- any untoward or significant patient reaction and its resolution.

*Rationale:*

According to AORN "Recommended practices for documentation of perioperative nursing care," documentation of patient care provides information for continuity of care, a mechanism for evaluating the effects of nursing interventions, information for quality assessment and improvement, and research.

*Interpretive statement 2:*

Nursing diagnoses applicable to the patient receiving IV conscious sedation may include potential for
- anxiety related to environment and procedure,
- ineffective breathing pattern or impaired gas exchange related to altered level of consciousness or airway obstruction,
- knowledge deficit related to poor recall,
- decreased cardiac output related to drug effect on myocardium, and
- injury related to altered level of consciousness.

*Rationale:*

Use of nursing diagnosis for planning the care of the patient receiving IV conscious sedation provides for patient-oriented care that focuses on the individual's response to the intervention. Nursing interventions are directed toward positive patient outcomes.

### Recommended Practice VI

**Patients receiving IV conscious sedation should be monitored postprocedure, receive written discharge instructions, and meet specified criteria before discharge.**

*Discussion:*

Postprocedure care, monitoring, and discharge criteria may vary depending on the type and amount of IV sedative administered, procedure performed, location and type of patient care unit, patient admission status (ie, inpatient or outpatient), and institutional policy. Hospitalized inpatients may require minimal recovery time, as they will continue to receive nursing care, while outpatients usually require a longer recovery time to return to a safe physiological level that will allow for discharge to home care.[16]

Patients and their families or significant others should receive written discharge instructions and verbalize an understanding of the instructions. Preprocedure and postprocedure instruction, as well as verbalization of understanding, is encouraged because at certain doses, drugs used for IV conscious sedation may cause amnesia, and patient recall may be affected.[17]

Discharge guidelines provide specific criteria for assessing and evaluating the patient's readiness for discharge and home care. Discharge criteria should reflect indicators that the patient has returned to a safe physiological level. These indicators may include vital signs, level of consciousness, mobility, airway patency, intact protective reflexes, skin color and condition, condition of dressing and surgical site, absence of protracted vomiting, and the ability to urinate. Presence of a responsible adult escort often is included as a necessary criterion for discharge. Discharge criteria should be developed by the medical staff of the institution in conjunction with the departments of anesthesia and nursing.

### Recommended Practice VII

**Policies and procedures on monitoring the patient receiving IV conscious sedation should be written, reviewed annually, and readily available within the practice setting.**

*Discussion:*

Policies and procedures for monitoring the patient receiving IV conscious sedation should include
- patient selection criteria,
- extent and responsibility for monitoring,
- method of recording patient data,
- frequency of the patient's physiological data documentation,
- medications that may be given by the registered nurse, and
- discharge criteria.

Policies and procedures are operational guidelines that are used to minimize risk factors, standardize practice, assist staff, and establish guidelines for quality assessment and improvement activities by establishing authority, responsibility, and accountability. Policies and procedures for monitoring the patient receiving IV conscious sedation also should be included in the orientation and ongoing education of all personnel in the practice setting.

*Source:* AORN Journal, April 1993, Vol. 54, # 3.

# Documentation of Perioperative Nursing Care

## Recommended Practice I

**The patient's record should reflect the perioperative plan of care including assessment, planning, implementation, evaluation, and expected outcome.**

*Interpretive statement 1:*
The patient's record should reflect the preoperative assessment performed by the perioperative nurse.

*Rationale:*
A documented assessment forms a baseline for planning care, continues through each subsequent phase, and provides for continuity of care.[1]

*Discussion:*
During the assessment process, the perioperative nurse collects data about the patient's status. Assessment is an ongoing process and should be done in accordance with the AORN "Standards of perioperative nursing practice."

*Interpretive statement 2:*
The patient's record should reflect the planning phase of care to be performed by the perioperative nurse.

*Rationale:*
Documentation of the planning phase should include the formulated goals and nursing strategies leading to desired patient outcomes.[2]

*Discussion:*
The planning phase begins when the perioperative nurse identifies nursing actions that will address the identified nursing diagnoses. The goal of these actions may be to prevent a potential patient problem or to intervene in an actual patient problem. Nursing diagnoses lead to the formulation of goals that represent desired patient outcomes.

*Interpretive statement 3:*
The patient's record should reflect nursing interventions provided during the perioperative phase of care.

*Rationale:*
Documentation of nursing interventions promotes continuity of care and improves communication among nursing personnel.[3]

*Discussion:*
The intervention phase depends on assessment and planning. Those activities determine what the nurse does to treat patient problems and to prevent potential problems from occurring.

*Interpretive statement 4:*
The patient's record should reflect continual evaluation of the perioperative nursing care and the patient's response to nursing interventions.

*Rationale:*
Documentation provides a mechanism for comparison of achieved patient goals to actual and expected patient outcomes.[4]

*Discussion:*
The nursing process requires that nurses evaluate how well the established patient goals were met and whether the activities of the perioperative nurse helped achieve those goals. Reassessment provides a measure for modifying the care plan. Documentation of patient outcomes also provides information for continuity of care, nursing quality assessment and improvement, perioperative nursing research, and risk management.

## Recommended Practice II

**Policies and procedures regarding documentation of perioperative nursing care should be written, reviewed annually, and readily available within the practice setting.**

*Discussion:*
The nursing process provides the governing framework for documenting perioperative nursing care. When nursing care is used in perioperative practice settings, it demonstrates the thoughts and actions taken by the nurse in the care of the surgical patient.[5]

Documentation should include information about the status of the patient, nursing interventions, the expected outcomes of perioperative nursing care, and the patient's response to that care.

The method of documenting perioperative nursing care may vary from one practice setting to another. The forms could include, but are not limited to, perioperative checklists, nurses' notes, flow sheets, care plans, and operative count records.[6]

# APPENDIX B — ASSOCIATION OF OPERATING ROOM NURSES RECOMMENDED PRACTICES

Every practice setting uses a formal system for documenting patient care. Records are different in each setting. The methods selected for documenting perioperative nursing care must fit with the institution's overall philosophy of nursing documentation and its system for record keeping. Perioperative documentation should include

- identification of persons providing care; name, title, and signature of the person responsible for the entry,
- evidence of a patient assessment upon arrival to the perioperative suite including the level of consciousness, psychosocial status, and baseline physical data,
- patient's overall skin condition on arrival and discharge from the perioperative suite,
- presence and disposition of sensory aids and prosthetic devices accompanying the patient to surgery. Prosthetic devices are defined as artificial substitutes for body parts (eg, arm, leg, eye, dentures, hearing aid, wig),
- patient's position, supports, and/or restraints used during the surgical procedure,
- placement of the dispersive electrode pad and identification of the electrosurgical unit and settings,
- placement of temperature control devices and identification of the unit recording time and temperature,
- placement of electrocardiographic or other monitoring electrodes,
- medications, irrigations, and solutions administered or dispensed by the registered nurse,
- specimens and cultures taken during the procedure,
- skin preparation, solutions, area prepared, and any reactions that may have occurred,
- placement of drains, catheters, packings, and dressings,
- placement of tourniquet cuff and person applying the cuff, pressure, time, and identification of the unit,
- urinary output and estimated blood loss, as appropriate,
- placement of implants (ie, tissue, inert or radioactive material inserted into a body cavity or grafted onto the tissue of the recipient), manufacturer, lot number, type, size, and other identifying information,
- occurrence and results of surgical item counts,
- time of discharge, disposition of patient, method of transfer, and patient status,
- intraoperative x-rays and flouroscopy,
- wound classification, and
- other direct patient care issues that are pertinent to patient outcomes.

These recommended practices should be used as guidelines for the development of policies and procedures for documentation within the practice setting. Policies and procedures establish authority, responsibility, and accountability, and serve as operational guidelines. An introduction and review of documentation policies and procedures should be included in the orientation and ongoing education of personnel to assist in the development of knowledge, skills, and attitudes that affect patient outcomes.

*Source:* AORN Journal, September, 1991, Vol. 57, # 4.

# APPENDIX C

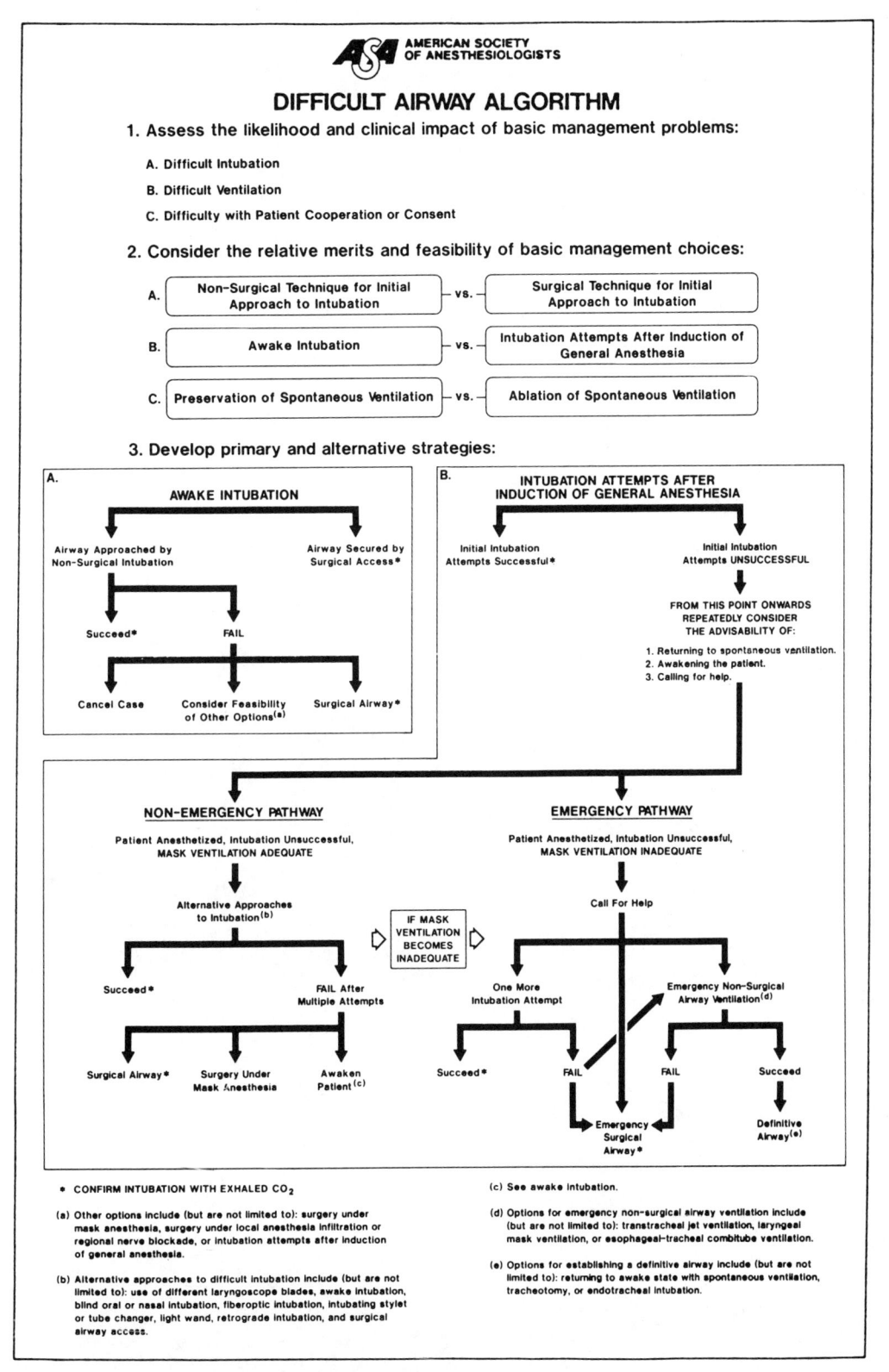

**AMERICAN SOCIETY OF ANESTHESIOLOGISTS**

## DIFFICULT AIRWAY ALGORITHM

1. Assess the likelihood and clinical impact of basic management problems:

    A. Difficult Intubation

    B. Difficult Ventilation

    C. Difficulty with Patient Cooperation or Consent

2. Consider the relative merits and feasibility of basic management choices:

    A. Non-Surgical Technique for Initial Approach to Intubation — vs. — Surgical Technique for Initial Approach to Intubation

    B. Awake Intubation — vs. — Intubation Attempts After Induction of General Anesthesia

    C. Preservation of Spontaneous Ventilation — vs. — Ablation of Spontaneous Ventilation

3. Develop primary and alternative strategies:

**A. AWAKE INTUBATION**
- Airway Approached by Non-Surgical Intubation
  - Succeed*
  - FAIL
    - Cancel Case
    - Consider Feasibility of Other Options[a]
    - Surgical Airway*
- Airway Secured by Surgical Access*

**B. INTUBATION ATTEMPTS AFTER INDUCTION OF GENERAL ANESTHESIA**
- Initial Intubation Attempts Successful*
- Initial Intubation Attempts UNSUCCESSFUL

FROM THIS POINT ONWARDS REPEATEDLY CONSIDER THE ADVISABILITY OF:
1. Returning to spontaneous ventilation.
2. Awakening the patient.
3. Calling for help.

**NON-EMERGENCY PATHWAY**
Patient Anesthetized, Intubation Unsuccessful, MASK VENTILATION ADEQUATE

Alternative Approaches to Intubation[b]
- Succeed*
- FAIL After Multiple Attempts
  - Surgical Airway*
  - Surgery Under Mask Anesthesia
  - Awaken Patient[c]

IF MASK VENTILATION BECOMES INADEQUATE →

**EMERGENCY PATHWAY**
Patient Anesthetized, Intubation Unsuccessful, MASK VENTILATION INADEQUATE

Call For Help

- One More Intubation Attempt
  - Succeed*
  - FAIL → Emergency Surgical Airway*
- Emergency Non-Surgical Airway Ventilation[d]
  - FAIL → Emergency Surgical Airway*
  - Succeed → Definitive Airway[e]

* CONFIRM INTUBATION WITH EXHALED $CO_2$

(a) Other options include (but are not limited to): surgery under mask anesthesia, surgery under local anesthesia infiltration or regional nerve blockade, or intubation attempts after induction of general anesthesia.

(b) Alternative approaches to difficult intubation include (but are not limited to): use of different laryngoscope blades, awake intubation, blind oral or nasal intubation, fiberoptic intubation, intubating stylet or tube changer, light wand, retrograde intubation, and surgical airway access.

(c) See awake intubation.

(d) Options for emergency non-surgical airway ventilation include (but are not limited to): transtracheal jet ventilation, laryngeal mask ventilation, or esophageal-tracheal combitube ventilation.

(e) Options for establishing a definitive airway include (but are not limited to): returning to awake state with spontaneous ventilation, tracheotomy, or endotracheal intubation.

*Source:* American Society of Anesthesiologists, Park Ridge, IL.

# BIBLIOGRAPHY

Acute Pain Management Guideline Panel. *Acute Pain Management: Operative or Medical Procedures and Trauma.* Clinical Practice Guideline. AHCPR Pub. No. 92-0032. Rockville, MD: Agency for Health Care Policy and Research, Public Health Service, U. S. Department of Health and Human Services. Feb. 1992.

Acute Pain Management Guideline Panel. *Acute Pain Management in Infants, Children and Adolescents: Operative and Medical Procedures. Quick Reference Guide for Clinicians.* AHCPR Pub. No. 92-0020. Rockville, MD: Agency for Health Care Policy and Research, Public Health Service, U. S. Department of Health and Human Services. Feb. 1992.

Association of Operating Room Nurses, Inc., (1993). Recommended practices: monitoring the patient receiving IV conscious sedation. *AORN J.*, 57:4.

Association of Operating Room Nurses, Inc., (1991). Recommended practices: documentaion of perioperative nursing care. *AORN J.*, 54:3.

Burden, N. (1993). *Ambulatory surgical nursing.* Philadelphia: W. B. Saunders.

Caldwell, L. M. (1991). Surgical outpatient concerns: what every perioperative nurse should know. *AORN J.*, 53:3.

Carmody, S., Hickey, P., Bookbinder, M. (1991). Perioperative needs of families. *AORN J.*, 54:3.

Cordell, B., Smith-Blair, N. (1994). Streamlined charting for patient education. *Nursing '94*, 24:1.

Donnelly, A. J. (1994). Malignant Hyperthermia: epidemiology, pathophysiology, treatment. *AORN J.*, 59:2.

Fraulini, K. E. (1987). *After anesthesia: a guide for PACU, ICU, and medical-surgical nurses.* Norwalk: Appleton & Lange.

Gay, C. R. (1990). The development of a postanesthesia record incorporating the nursing process. *J. Post Anesthesia Nursing*, 5:2.

Gruendemann, B. J., & Meeker, M. H. (1987). *Alexander's care of the patient in surgery.* St. Louis: C. V. Mosby.

Gulczynski, D. (1993). "Production pressure" danger avoided by CQI effort. *Anesthesia Patient Safety Foundation Newsletter*, 8:3.

Hardick, M., ed. (1989). *Manual of Gastrointestinal Procedures, 2nd ed.* New York: Society of Gastroenterology Nurses and Associates, Inc.

Leino-Kilpi, H., & Buorenheimo, J. (1993). Perioperative nursing care quality: patients' opinions. *AORN J.*, 57:5.

Kemmy, J. A. (1993). OR Nursing Law: Legal implications of perioperative documentaion. *AORN J.* 57:4.

Llewellyn, J. G. (1991). Short stay surgery: present practices, future trends. *AORN J.* 53:5.

Maltby, J.R., Sutherland A.D., Sale J.P., et al (1986): Preoperative oral fluidsis a five-hour fast justified prior to elective surgery? *Anesth. Analg.*, 65:1112.

McCorkmick, R. M., Gilson-Parkevich, T. (1976). *Patient and family education: tools, techniques, and theory.* New York: John Wiley & Sons.

McCarr, J. (1992). Chemo patients' surprise: they're hungry! *Hospital Pharmacist Report*, December.

Miller, R. A., ed. (1990). *Anesthesia, 3rd ed.* Philadelphia: W. B. Saunders Company.

Murphy, E. K. (1993). OR nursing law: Patients deserve respectful surgical environment. *AORN J.*, 57:5.

Rogers, A., Rosas, J., O'Hanlon-Nichols, T. (1994). How to inject a subcutaneous abdominal implant. *Nursing '94*, 42:1.

Shafer, S. L. (1993). Advances in propofol pharmacokinetics and pharmacodynamics. *J. Clin. Anesth.* 5(Suppl 1): 14S-21S.

Sheperd, S. (1990). Helping ambulatory surgery patients cope with emotions. *J. Postanesthesia Nsg.*, 5:2.

Sparks, S. M. & Taylor, C. M. (1991). *Nursing diagnosis reference manual: an indispensable guide to better patient care.* Springhouse PA: Springhouse Corporation.

Steelman, V. M. (1990). Intraoperative music therapy: effects on anxiety, blood pressure. *AORN J.* 52:5.

Tatum, P. L., & Defalque, R. J. (1994). Subarachnoid injection during retrobulbar block: a case report. *J. of American Association of Nurse Anesthetists*, 62:1.

White, P.F., Vasconez, L.O., Mathes, S., et al. (1988). Comparison of midazolam and diazepam for sedation during plastic surgery. *J. Plast. Reconstr. Surg.* 81:703.

Yale, E. (1993). Preoperative teaching strategy. *AORN J.* 57:4.

# SUGGESTED READING

Acute Pain Management Guideline Panel. *Acute Pain Management: Operative or Medical Procedures and Trauma.* Clinical Practice Guideline. AHCPR Pub. No. 92-0032. Rockville, MD: Agency for Health Care Policy and Research, Public Health Service, U. S. Department of Health and Human Services. Feb. 1992. Call (800) 358-9295 for copy.

Acute Pain Management Guideline Panel. *Acute Pain Management in Infants, Children and Adolescents: Operative and Medical Procedures. Quick Reference Guide for Clinicians.* AHCPR Pub. No. 92-0020. Rockville, MD: Agency for Health Care Policy and Research, Public Health Service, U. S. Department of Health and Human Services. Feb. 1992. Call (800) 358-9295 for copy.

Beck, C. F. Malignant hyperthermia: are you prepared? *AORN J.*, 59:2, 367-389. *Excellent article with up-to-date information.*

Burden, N. (1993). *Ambulatory surgical nursing.* Philadelphia: W. B. Saunders. *Well written, this book is an invaluable resource for ambulatory nurses; ambulatory units might want to keep a copy on hand for reference.*

Gay, C. R. (1990). The development of a postanesthesia record incorporating the nursing process. *J. of Post Anesthesia Nursing,* 5:2. *Good article about applying the nursing process; includes a well designed PACU record.*

Hardick, M., ed. (1989). *Manual of Gastrointestinal Procedures, 2nd ed.* New York: Society of Gastroenterology Nurses and Associates, Inc. *Excellent reference by nurses, for nurses.*

Kidwell, J. A. (1991). Nursing care for the patient receiving conscious sedation during gastrointestinal endoscopic procedures. *Gastroenterolody Nursing,* 14:3, p. 134-139. *Good article focusing on nursing concerns.*

Llewellyn, J. G. (1993). Short stay surgery: present practices, future trends. *AORN J.* 53: 5, p. 1179-1191. *Good review article.*

Lippincott Manual of Nursing Practice, 4th ed. (1986). Chapter 2, Health Education and the Nursing Process. Philadelphia: Lippincott. *A concise review of principles of teaching and learning, this brief chapter integrates patient teaching with the nursing process.*

Murphy, D. (1993). Managing patient stress in endoscopy. *Gastroenterology Nursing,* 16:2, 72-74. *A discussion of non-pharmacologic stress reduction methods.*

# GLOSSARY

**ABC:** Acronym for airway, breathing, and circulation—or: the first priority in caring for any patient.

**Abdominoplasty:** Surgical revision and restructuring of the appearance of the abdomen; usually performed by a plastic surgeon.

**Abortion**: Termination of pregnancy. Abortion may be spontaneeous and is usually called a "miscarriage" by the layperson in this case. Abortion may also be elective.

**Adhesions:** Scar tissue that forms around areas of previous tissue damage such as from surgery, inflammation, or pathology. Adhesions are commonly associated with abdominal and gynecologic surgery and can cause pain, infertility, and intestinal obstruction.

**Analgesia**: Relief from pain or reduction in pain.

**Anesthesia:** Loss of sensation producing insensitivity to pain.

**Anesthesiologist:** A physician who administers anesthesia; may or may not be board-certified in anesthesia, although many institutions are moving towards this requirement.

**Arthroplasty:** Surgical revision of joint; an example is correction of hammertoes.

**Arthroscopy:** Use of a lighted instrument to visualize the inside of a joint.

**Arthrotomy:** Incision of a joint.

**ASA Physical Status (PS):** A classification system developed by the American Society of Anesthesiologists that ranks patients from PS 1 to PS 6, with PS 1 being a healthy patient; PS 5 a moribund patient, and PS 6 a brain dead patient. Higher numbers indicate greater risk of morbidity and mortality during surgery and anesthesia.

**Aspiration pneumonia:** A type of pneumonia that results from inhaling gastric contents.

**Aspiration prophylaxis:** One or more drugs that may be administered to increase the pH of the gastric contents and hasten emptying or the stomach; goal is to reduce the chance of aspiration and minimize damage to the lungs in the event aspiration does occur.

**Augmentation mammoplasty:** An aesthetic procedure invoving placement of artificial implants for the purpose of increasing the size of the breasts.

**Bartholin's cyst**: A cyst of the female genital tract.

**Benzodiazepines:** A class of tranquilizers that include diazepam (Valium) and midazolam (Versed), which is popular in ambulatory care because of its shortened duration of action. Contraindicated during pregnancy because of possible teratogenic effects.

**Biopsy:** Removal of a tissue specimen from the body for the purpose of examining for pathology or study.

**Blepharoplasty:** Surgical revision of the eyelids; often performed by a plastic surgeon.

**Bronchoscopy:** Use of a lighted instrument to visualize inside the tracheobronchial tree.

**Bunionectomy:** Excision of a bunion, which is an inflammation and swelling of the bursa at the great toe.

**Cardioversion:** Application of an electrical charge to the heart to convert an arrhythmia to normal sinus rthym.

**Carpal tunnel release:** Surgical procedure performed to release constricting tissue around the median nerve in the hand and wrist.

**Catecholamines:** Hormones released in response to stress; part of the body's "fight or flight" mechanism. Catecholamines raise the blood pressure, elevate the heart rate, and release sugar into the bloodstream among other effects.

**Cerebrospinal fluid:** Fluid that bathes the spinal cord and brain, providing a protective cushion and barrier. It is normally clear and straw-colored.

**Cervix:** The lower part or neck of the uterus.

**Cervical dysplasia:** Abnormal cells in the cervix; often detected by a Pap smear.

**Cervical conization:** Excision of a tissue sample from the cervix.

**Chemotherapy:** Administration of drugs developed to fight illness; often used to refer to agents used to battle cancer.

**Chorionic villus sampling (CVS):** A genetic screening test for abnormalities in the developing fetus. Performed on an ambulatory basis in the first trimester.

**Colonoscopy:** Use of a lighted instrument to visualize the inside of the colon.

**Cornea:** The clear portion of the sclera at the front of the eye.

**CPR:** Acronym for cardiopulmonary resuscitation; all nurses should be trained in basic CPR skills.

**Cricothyroidotomy:** Puncture of the cricothyroid membrane in order to deliver oxygen to the lungs. Generally performed as an emergency airway access technique when other conventional methods at tracheal intubation have failed.

**Cricoid pressure:** Compression of the cricoid cartilage in the neck; performed by an assistant during endotracheal intubation to reduce the potential for stomach contents to be inhaled during intubation.

**CRNA (Certified Registered Nurse Anesthetist):** An RN with advanced, accredited training and national professional board certification in the administration of anesthesia.

**Cryotherapy:** Freezing abnormal cells to destroy them; often a gynecologic procedure performed on the cervix.

**Cyst:** A fluid or semi-liquid filled tissue sac.

**Cystoscopy:** Use of a lighted instrument to visualize the inside of the bladder.

**D & C:** Dilation and curettage; refers to a surgical procedure (diagnostic or therapeutic) that involves dilating the cervix and then scraping the inside of the uterus. Performed for dysfunctional uterine bleeding and other gynecologic disorders.

**Dura:** Toughest and outermost of the meninges or tissues that cover the brain and spinal cord. The dura is deliberately punctured to administer spinal anesthesia.

**Electroconvulsive therapy (ECT):** Shock treatment; temporarily triggers a seizure. Used as treatment of psychiatric disorders such as depression; often performed in the postanesthesia care unit (PACU).

**Endometrial ablation:** A surgical procedure to destroy the lining of the uterus; indicated to relieve dysfunctional uterine bleeding, most often in women who desire no more children, because it generally results in permanent infertility.

**Endometriosis:** An abnormal condition in which the lining of the uterus (endometrium) grows outside of the uterus, often around the ovaries and tubes; can cause pain and infertility.

**Endoscopy:** Use of a lighted instrument to visualize the inside of a body cavity; often refers to the visualization of the inside of the upper GI tract.

**Endoscopic Retrograde Cholangiopancreatography (ERCP):** Use of a lighted instrument to identify injection sites that will enable the physician to visualize the pancreatic and biliary ducts and inject dye for the purpose of obtaining x-ray films. The duodenoscope is passed through the mouth and into the duodenum.

**Endotracheal intubation:** Placement of a breathing tube into the trachea (windpipe); usually accomplished with the aid of a metal instrument called a largyngoscope.

**Epidural anesthesia:** Above the dura, which covers the spinal cord, lies the epidural space. Local anesthetic (LA) can be injected into this space to induce analgesia and anesthesia. The epidural technique may be continuous, so more LA can be injected as necessary.

**Esophagoscopy:** Use of a lighted instrument to visualize the inside of the esophagus.

**Gastroscopy:** Use of a lighted instrument to visualize the inside of the stomach.

**General anesthesia:** A state of unconsciousness characterized by muscle relaxation, amnesia, and analgesia.

**Globe:** The eyeball.

**Hemostasis:** To stop bleeding, as during surgery.

**Hymenectomy/hymenotomy:** Surgical procedure performed on an ambulatory basis to release the hymen, which is tissue that can cover the introitus or opening to the vagina.

**Hypovolemic shock:** Lowered blood pressure resulting from inadequate volume of blood for the heart to pump through the body; may result from excessive bleeding and insufficient fluid replacement during surgery.

**Hysterectomy:** Removal of the uterus through the vagina or the abdomen; vaginal hysterectomy may be performed on an ambulatory basis in selected patients; abdominal hysterectomy generally requires hospitalization or short stay programs.

**Hysteroscopy:** Visualization of the uterine cavity by means of a lighted instrument (hysteroscope).

**Inhalation anesthetic agents:** Liquids that are heated to the vapor state by the anesthesia machine and delivered to the patient's lungs in a carrier gas such as oxygen. Once in the lungs, the agent is circulated to the brain, where it causes unconsciousness. There are currently four inhalation agents: isoflurane, fluothane, and enflurane; a new agent known as desflurane (Suprane) was recently introduced and should find popularity in ambulatory surgery.

**Intravenous regional anesthesia:** A technique that involves exsanguinating and occluding the circulation of the extremity and filling the veins with local anesthetic; commonly used for soft tissue procedures on hands or feet. Also known as a Bier block.

**Laparoscopy:** Visualization of the internal pelvic structures by means of a lighted instrument (laparoscope).

**Laryngoscopy:** Use of a lighted instrument to visualize the larynx.

**Laser:** An instrument that concentrates heat and light into a form that can be used to manipulate tissue, usually by burning and destroying. Used in ambulatory surgery to destroy abnormal tissue such as pelvic adhesions or genital warts.

**Ligament:** Fibrous tissue that connects bone to bone; torn ligaments are often repaired on an ambulatory basis.

**Lipectomy:** Surgical removal of fatty tissue; often aided by powerful suction and performed as an ambulatory procedure.

**Mammogram:** A special x-ray for detection of pathology in the breasts.

**Manual ventilating bag:** A bag-valve-mask system; consists of a pliable reservoir connected to an oxygen source and a coupling that adapts to an endotracheal tube or a mask. Used to manually ventilate a patient whose respiratory efforts are inadequate or one who is apneic.

**Myringotomy:** Incision of the tympanic membrane.

**Neuromuscular blocking agents:** Drugs that block transmission of impulses at the neuromuscular junction and therefore paralyze the patient.

**Oculocardiac reflex:** Sudden bradycardia or asystole; results from traction on the eye muscles or pressure on the globe and is usually relieved when the stimulus is halted.

**Oophorectomy:** Surgical removal of the ovary.

**Otoplasty:** Plastic surgical revision of the ear.

**Pap smear:** An early screening test for cancer and other pathology in the female; involves scraping cells from the cervix for examination under the microscope.

**Pharynx:** The muscular structure known as the throat; serves as part of the upper airway and also as a passageway for food.

**Regional anesthesia:** Inducing a state of insensitivity to pain (anesthesia) by injecting local anesthetics (LA) into a specific area of the body. Common types of RA include: Spinal, Epidural, and Intravenous Regional or Bier Block, and nerve blocks. Often simply referred to as a block.

**Retrobulbar block:** A technique of injecting LA around the globe of the eye to produce anesthesia; often used in cataract surgery.

**Rhinoplasty:** Surgical revision and reshaping of the nose; often performed by a plastic surgeon.

**Rhytidectomy:** Face lift.

**Salpingectomy:** Removal of the fallopian tubes.

**Septoplasty:** Surgical revision of the septum in the nose.

**Sigmoidoscopy:** Use of a lighted instrument to visualize the inside of the sigmoid colon; may be performed in a doctor's office.

**Spinal anesthesia:** Also known as a subarchnoid block. The dura, or covering of the spinal cord is pierced with a slender needle, and a local anesthetic is deposited in the CSF.

**Tamponade:** Pressure or compression.

**Tarsal tunnel release:** Surgical release of constricting tissue in the foot.

**Tendon:** Fibrous tissue that connects muscle to bone; repairs are often performed on an ambulatory basis.

**Trachea:** A hollow tube, composed of rings, that serves as the air passage from the throat to the lungs; obstruction quickly results in death.

**Tubal ligation:** A permanent method of inducing sterility in the female by interrupting the fallopian tubes; may be accomplished with cutting, burning, and application of rings. Commonly performed on an ambulatory basis but does not guarantee sterility. Reversal is difficult and not always successful.

**Ureters:** Muscular tubes that carry urine from the kidneys to the bladder.

**Urethra:** The duct that carries urine from the body after collection in the bladder.

**Uterus:** A female reproductive organ, also called the "womb" by laypeople.

**Vagina:** Part of the female reproductive tract, forms a passageway from the uterus to the outside of the body; distensible and elastic before menopause.

**Vasectomy:** Severing of the vas deferens in the male reproductive system to induce permanent sterility, although failure of the technique is possible. Usually performed with local anesthesia on an ambulatory basis.

**Vasovasotomy:** Reversal of vasectomy for the purpose of restoring male fertility; usually performed on ambulatory basis in a procedure lasting 2-4 hours.

# INDEX

## A

Abnormal pseudocholinesterase level, 70
Accreditation Association for Ambulatory Health Care, 12
Admission,
    perioperative, 64
    to operating room (OR), 81
    to PACU, 97
Adriamycin, 162
Advance Directive Notification, 21
Agonist-antagonist agents,
    as preanesthesia medication, 73
    used during anesthesia, 36–38
Air, 41
Airway,
    compromise of, 168–170
    maintaining patient, 98
    surgical manipulation of the, 140
Alfenta, 37
Alfentanil (Alfenta), 37
Allergies, 65
Ambu bag, 159
Ambulatory care,
    advantages and disadvantages of, 3–4
    alternatives to, 4–5
    development of, 2–3
    during procedure, 79–90
    during regional/local anesthesia or conscious sedation, 49–59
    facilities for, 9–14
    following procedure, 93–104
    future of, 5
    general anesthesia considerations in, 31–46
    nursing process and, 18–20
    preparing patient for procedures of, 61–76
    selecting patient for, 25–29
    special considerations of, 20–21
    See also Procedures; Surgical specialties
Ambulatory record (sample), 66
Ambulatory surgery, 130
    See also Surgical specialties
American College of Radiology, 12
American Nurses Association, 55
American Society of Anesthesiologists PS classifications, 26–27
Amidate, 38
Amniocentesis, 159
Ancillary personnel, 63
Anectine, 39
Anesthesia care plan, 71
    See also General anesthesia
Anesthesia team, 63
Anesthesiologists, 63
Anesthetic emergencies,
    airway compromise as, 168–170
    cardiovascular compromise as, 170
    malignant hyperthermia as, 171
Angiography, 158
Angioplasty, 158
Antagonists, 86
Antibiotics, 73
Antibiotic therapy, 162
Anticholinergics, 72–73
Antiemetics, 73
Anti-inflammatory ketorolac (Toradol), 137
Antilirium, 99
Anxiety,
    of cardiology patients, 159
    over genetic testing, 160
    patient, 57
Arrhythmias, 170, 173
Arteriograms, 156
Arthroscopic procedures, 135
Arthrotomy, 135
Asepsis, 80
Aspiration, 170, 172
Aspiration pneumonitis, 34–35
Assessment,
    discharge, 108
    patient, 18
    perioperative, 63–68
    preanesthesia, 69–71
    See also Nursing strategies
Association of Operating Room Nurses (AORN), 55
Ateriograms, 157
Atropine, 39

## B

Barbiturates,
    as preanesthesia medication, 72
    used during anesthesia, 36, 38
Bicitra, 170
Bier Block, 53

Biopsy, 163
Bladder distention, 104
Blenoxane, 162
Bleomycin (Blenoxane), 162
Blood pressure, 42
Blood products, 162, 174
Bone marrow aspiration, 163
Breath sounds, 42
Bronchoscopy, 164
Bupivacaine (Marcaine), 54
Butorphanol (Stadol), 37
Butterworth Hospital, 2
Butyrophenone droperidol (Inaspine), 37

## C

Cardiac arrest, 173
Cardiac catheterization, 158
Cardiac procedures, 157–159
Cardiovascular compromise, 170
Cardiovascular surgery, 147
Cardioversion, 158
Carrier gases, 41
Cataract extraction, 145
Catecholamine (stress hormones) release, 33
Cerebrospinal fluid (CSF), 51–52
Certified Registered Nurse Anesthetists (CRNA), 63
Cervical procedures, 132
Chemotherapy, 161
Chloroprocaine (Nesacaine), 54
Chorionic villus sampling (CVS), 160
Cocaine, 54
Colonoscopy, 152
"Come and Go" Surgery Unit (George Washington University), 2
Complications,
  delaying discharge, 108
  due to arthroscopic procedures, 135
  due to cervical/vaginal procedures, 132
  due to ear procedures, 140
  due to genitalia procedures, 132
  due to intra-abdominal surgery, 131
  due to intra-uterine procedures, 131–132
  due to nose/sinus procedures, 140
  due to ophthalmic surgery, 145
  due to oral surgery, 141
  due to plastic surgery, 138
  due to throat procedures, 140
  due to urologic surgery, 143
  postanesthesia, 97, 99
  support person in case of, 110
Computer-assisted scans (CAT scans), 156
Conscious sedation,
  described, 55–56
  nursing strategies for, 56–59
Contact lenses, 76
Crash (code) cart, 103, 123
Cytotoxic anticancer drugs, 162

## D

Dantrolene (Dantrium), 171
Desflurane (Suprane), 40–41, 94
Diagnosis,
  of ambulatory patient, 18–19
  during regional/local anesthesia or conscious sedation, 57
  for ENT or oral surgery patient, 142
  for gastrointestinal procedures, 152–154
  for gynecologic patient, 133
  for ophthalmic surgery patient, 146
  for orthopedic patient, 136
  for patient preparing for discharge, 111
  for patients preparing for procedure, 67
  for patients with surgical emergencies, 169
  for patients undergoing general anesthesia, 44
  perioperative assessment leading to, 68
  for plastic surgery patient, 139
  postanesthesia, 96
  *See also* Nursing strategies
Dialysis, 163
Diazepam (Valium), 37, 39, 73
Diet, discharge instructions on, 110–111
Difficult intubation, 169–170, 172
Diprivan, 33, 38, 45, 94, 161
Discharge,
  from postanesthesia room, 99, 101
  instructions for geriatric patients, 122
  instructions given during, 110–112
  instructions for pediatric patients, 120
  recovery phase 2 prior to, 107–108
Discharge Criteria Form, 109
Dissociative agent, 36, 38–39
Documentation,
  discharge, 115
  facility, 69
  operative, 82
  PACU, 99
Doxorubicin (Adriamycin), 162
Droperidol (Inapsine), 99
Duragesic, 115

## E

Ear procedures, 139–140
Echocardiogram, 157
Electrocardiograms (ECG), 41, 157
Electrocautery, 153
Electroconvulsive therapy (ECT), 163
Emergence delirium, 99
Emergency patients, 123, 126
EMLA, 118–119
Endoscope, 152
Endoscopic retrograde cholangiopancreatography (ERCP), 153
End-tidal CO2 monitor, 41–42
Enflurane (Ethrane), 40
ENT surgery, 138–143
Environment,
  ambience of patient, 81
  facility, 12–13
  procedure suite, 80–81
Epidural, 163
Epidural anesthesia and analgesia (EA), 52–53, 94–95
Equipment (procedure suite), 80
Esophageal dilatation, 153
Esophagogastroduodenoscopy (EGD), 152
Etomidate (Amidate), 38
Eutetic mixture os local anesthetics (EMLA), 118–119
Exercise treadmill test, 157–158
Extracorporeal shock-wave lithotripsy (ESWL), 143
Extraocular procedures, 145

## F

Facilities,
  accommodating parents with pediatric patients, 119
  development of assisted-care, 4–5
  disaster preparation within, 13
  documentation in, 69
  environment of, 12–13
  evaluation of, 3
  patient preparation within, 62
  security measures within, 13
  standard of care in, 12, 21
  types of ambulatory care, 9–12
Families,
  anesthesia history within, 70
  as patient support system, 82, 85
  postanesthesia support of, 99
  preoperative and preprocedure teaching for, 68–69
  separation of pediatric patients from, 119
  *See also* Support system
Fasting requirements,
  described, 34–35
  for pediatric patients, 118
  *See also* General anesthesia
Fentanyl (Sublimaze), 37, 86, 118
Fentanyl transfermal system (Duragesic), 115
Filtration masks, 87
Flexible sigmoidoscopy, 153
Fluid balance, 119, 123
Flumazenil (Romazicon), 37, 86
Fluothane, 40
Follow-up care, 112
Follow-up Record, 113
Forane, 40
Freestanding ambulatory units, 11

## G

Gastrointestinal (GI) procedures, 152–154
General anesthesia,
  airway compromise during, 168–170
  cardiovascular compromise during, 170
  contraindications to, 34–35
  for geriatric patients, 122
  inhalation agents used in, 40–41
  intravenous agents used during, 35–40
  Malignant Hyperthermia (MH) during, 171
  monitoring patient under, 41–42, 82
  nursing for patient undergoing, 42–45, 85–89
  patient monitors used in, 43
  for pediatric patients, 118–119
  preanesthesia evaluation, 69–71
  preanesthesia medication, 71–73
  process of, 32–34
  recovery from, 94
  *See also* Local anesthesia (LA); Regional anesthesia
General surgery, 147
Genitalia procedures, 132
Geriatric patients, 120–122, 125
Goserelin acetate implant (Zoladex), 161
Gynecology surgery, 130–134

## H

Haloperidol (Haldol), 37
Halothane (Fluothane), 40
Heart sounds, 42

Holter ECG monitoring, 157
Hospitals, 10–11
Hydration, 163
Hypnotic agents (non-narcotic/barbiturate), 36, 38
Hypotension, 108, 114, 173
Hypothermia, 99, 119

# I

Impaired patients, 122–123, 125
Inapsine, 37, 99
Inhalation agents, 40–41
Injected intravenously (IV), 32–33
Inspired oxygen, 42
Insurance companies,
   facilities paid for by, 9–10
   patient decisions made by, 28
Intercostal block, 163–164
Intra-abdominal surgery, 131
Intraocular procedures, 145
Intraoperative awareness, 88
Intra-uterine procedures, 131–132
Intravenous(IV) fluids, 123, 168
Intravenous regional anesthesia, 53, 95
Isoflurane (Forane), 40
IV dipyridamole (Persantine) thallium test, 158

# J

Jehovah's Witnesses, 174
Joint Commission for Accreditation of Health Care Organizations, 12
Joint Commission on Accreditation of Hospitals, 68

# K

Ketamine (Ketalar), 38–39, 118

# L

Laparoscopy, 131, 134
Laryngectomy, 140
Laryngospasm, 168–169
Laughing gas, 37, 41
Legal issues, 21
Lidocaine (Xylocaine), 54, 95
Lithotripsy, 143
Local anesthesia (LA),
   described, 54–55
   monitoring, 55–56
   nursing strategies during, 56–59
   recovery from, 95

used for spinal anesthesia, 51–52
*See also* General anesthesia; Regional anesthesia

# M

Magnetic resonance imaging (MRI), 135, 156, 157
Malignant Hyperthermia (MH), 70, 171, 173
*Manual of Gastrointestinal Procedures,* 152
Marcaine, 54
Medications,
   discharge instructions regarding, 110
   preanesthesia, 71–73
   taken by geriatric patients, 122
Metoclopramide (Reglan), 99, 170
Midazolam (Versed), 37, 86, 118
Monitored anesthesia care (MAC), 55, 69, 119
Morphine, 86
"Muscle relaxants," 39–40

# N

Nalbuphine (Nubain), 37
Naloxone (Narcan), 37, 38, 86
Narcotics,
   as preanesthesia medication, 73
   used during anesthesia, 35–37
Nausea and vomiting (N & V),
   antiemetics for, 73
   discharge delayed due to, 108
   during previous anesthetic experiences, 70
   NPO to reduce, 75
   postanesthesia, 99
   triggered by other recovering patients, 104
Nerve blocks, 53–54, 95, 163–164
Nerve stimulator, 42
Nesacaine, 54
Neuromuscular blocking agents, 36, 39–40
Neurovascular compromise, 135
Nicotine transdermal patch, 75
Nitrous oxide (laughing gas), 37, 41
Nonstress test, 160
Norcuron, 39
North American Nursing Diagnosis Association (NANDA), 18
Nose procedures, 140
NPO, 65, 75, 81, 118
Nubain, 37
Nurse anesthetist, 63
Nurse Practice Act, 85, 112
Nurses,
   ambulatory care expectations of, 5
   care freestanding units by, 11

care in hospitals by, 10–11
care in physician offices by, 12
documentation by, 69
influence on patient care by, 28–29
legal considerations for, 21
as part of periorperative team, 63
preanesthesia interview by, 70–71
precautions in handling cytotoxic anticancer drugs for, 162
responsibilities of surgery, 20
teaching patients, 20, 69
Nursing strategies,
assessment, 18
for chemotherapy patient, 161–162
during discharge, 112, 113–115
during preoperative patient preparation, 68, 73–76
during procedure, 85–89
during surgical/anesthetic emergencies, 171–174
or ENT patient, 141–143
evaluation of care, 19–20
for gynecologic patient, 132–134
implementation of care, 19
for obstetric patient, 160
for ophthalmic surgery patient, 145–147
for orthopedic patient, 135–137
for patient receiving blood products, 162
for patient with special needs, 123–126
for patient under general anesthesia, 42–45
for patient undergoing cardiac procedures, 159
for patient undergoing GI procedures, 154
for patient undergoing radiologic procedures, 156–157
planning care, 19
for plastic surgery patient, 138
for postanesthesia care, 101–104
for urologic surgery patient, 143–145
*See also* Diagnosis

## O

Obstetrical procedures, 159–160
Obstetric surgery, 130–134
Oculocardiac reflex, 145
Ondansetron (Zofran), 99, 161
Operative site, 82
Ophthalmic surgery, 145–147
Opioid analgesics, 35–37
Oral intake, 65
Oral surgery, 138–143
Orthopedic procedures, 134–137
Otolaryngology (ENT) surgery, 138–143
Outpatient Clinic (UCLA), 2
Oxygen, 41, 85, 89
Oxytocin challenge test, 160

## P

PACU, 94–95, 97, 99
Pain,
cautionary use of duragesic for, 115
as complication, 97, 99
discharge delayed by, 108
management of, 163–164
management of pediatric patient, 119–120
postoperative phase of, 102
preventing/relieving postoperative, 100–101
Pancuronium (Pavulon), 39
Pap smear, 130
Parenteral therapy, 161–162
Patients,
age of, 26, 34
ambulatory pediatric, 118–120
ambulatory procedure preparation for, 61–76
assessment of, 18
care during procedure of, 85–90
care environment for, 12–13
considering procedures performed on, 27
development of services for, 2–3
diagnosis of, 18–19
discharging the, 107–115
emergence delirium of, 99
general anesthesia monitors for, 43
general anesthesia used on ambulatory, 32–35
geriatric, 120–122, 125
health status (PS classifications) of, 26–27
height/weight, 65
impaired, 122–123, 125
influence of nurses on care of, 28–29
legal considerations for, 21
monitoring while under anesthesia, 41–42, 82
pediatric, 118–120, 123–125
perioperative assessment, 63–68
physical exam of, 65, 68
physician decisions for, 28
positioning, 81–82
postanesthesia care of, 93–104
preanesthesia evaluation of, 69–71

refusing blood products, 174
regional/local anesthesia or conscious sedation of, 49–59
rights and responsibilities of, 21
security measures for, 13
strategies for gynecologic, 132–134
teaching, 20, 69
third-party payer decisions for, 28
trauma and emergency, 123, 126
using regional/local anesthesia on, 49–59
*See also* Surgical specialties
Pediatric crash (code) cart, 123
Pediatric patients, 118–120, 123–125
Pelvic exam, 130
"Pelvic rest," 134
Pentothal, 33
Percutaneous endoscopic gastrostomy (PEG), 153–154
Percutaneous liver biopsy, 153
Perioperative assessment/planning,
  baseline vital signs taken for, 68
  described, 63–64
  documentation of, 82
  family/patient teaching during, 68–69
  listing all current medications, 64
  listing allergies, 65
  nursing strategies during, 73–76
  patient emotional status, 65
  patient height/weight, 65
  physical exam of patient, 65, 68
  preanesthesia evaluation during, 69–71
  preanesthesia medications, 71–73
  reason for admission part of, 64
  recording presence of prosthetics, 65
  reviewing body systems/health status part of, 64
  sample ambulatory record, 66
  taking social history, 65
  time of last oral intake, 65
Persantine thallium test, 158
PET scans, 156
Physical activities, 111
Physical examination, 71
Physicians,
  care in offices of, 11–12
  explanations to families by, 68
  follow-up by, 110
  as part of perioperative team, 63
  patient consultation prior to anesthesia, 87
  patient decisions made by, 28
Physostigmine (Antilirium), 99

Plastic surgery, 137–138
Pneumatic tourniquet (TQ), 53, 134–135
Podiatry procedures, 134–137
Positioning (patient), 81–82
Postanesthesia care, 95–101
Postanesthesia care unit (PACU), 94–95, 97, 99
Postprocedure Instruction Sheet, 155
Preanesthesia evaluation, 69–71
Preanesthesia medication, 71–73
Preanesthesia tests, 35
Procedures,
  discharge from, 85
  documentation of, 82
  general anesthesia during, 32–35
  nursing responsibilities during, 20
  nursing strategies during, 85–89
  for pediatric patients, 118–120
  periorperative team listed, 62–63
  postanesthesia care following, 95–101
  preparing patient in ambulatory setting for, 62
  preparing procedure suite for, 80–81, 82
  using regional anesthesia, 50–51
  *See also* Surgical specialties; Therapeutic procedures
Propofol (Diprivan), 33, 38, 45, 94, 161
Prosthetics, 65, 71, 76
PS classifications, 26–27
Pulmonary function studies, 164
Pulse oximeter, 42, 85

# R

Radiation therapy, 156
Radiologic procedures, 154, 156–157
Ranitidine (Zantac), 170
Recovery phase 2, 107–108
Regional anesthesia,
  indications for, 50–51
  intravenous, 53
  recovery from, 94–95
  using epidural anesthesia and analgesia, 52–53
  using nerve blocks, 53–54
  using spinal anesthesia, 51–52
  *See also* General anesthesia; Local anesthesia (LA)
Reglan, 99, 170
Romazicon, 37, 86

# S

Sclerotherapy, 153
Secobarbital (Seconal), 38

Seconal, 38
"Short stay" surgery, 4
Sinus procedures, 140
"Skillful neglect," 103
Smoking, 75, 138
Sodium citrate (Bicitra), 170
Sodium pentothal (Thiopental), 38
Sodium thiopental (Pentothal), 33
Sonogram, 160
Spinal anesthesia, 51–52, 94
Stadol, 37
Stellate ganglion, 163
"Straight local," 54
Subarachnoid block (SAB), 51–52
Sublimaze, 37, 86, 118
Succinylcholine (Anectine), 39
Sufentanil (Sufenta), 118
Supplies (procedure suite), 80–81
Support system, 68–69, 99, 110
    See also Families
Suprane, 40–41, 94
Surgical emergencies, 168
Surgical specialties,
    ambulatory surgery, 130
    cardiovascular surgery, 147
    general surgery, 147
    gynecology and obstetrics, 130–134
    ophthalmic surgery, 145–147
    orthopedics and podiatry, 134–137
    otolaryngology and oral surgery, 138–143
    plastic surgery, 137–138
    urologic surgery, 143–145
    See also Ambulatory care; Procedures
Surgical technology, 2–3
Syncope, 108

# T

Technical surgical errors, 168
Temperature,
    patient, 42
    of procedure suite, 80
Therapeutic procedures,
    cardiac, 158
    described, 152
    gastrointestinal, 153–154
    obstetrical, 159–160
    pain management for, 163–164
    parenteral therapy as, 161–162
    pulmonary, 164

    radiologic, 156
    See also Procedures
Thermoregulation, 119
Thiopental, 38
Third-party payer. See Insurance companies
Throat procedures, 140
Tinnitus, 137
Toradol, 137
Total intravenous anesthesia (TIVA), 32–33
Tranquilizers,
    as preanesthesia medication, 72–73
    used during anesthesia, 36–37
Transdermal scopolamine patches (Trans-derm Scop), 99
Transesophageal echocardiography (TEE), 158
Trauma patients, 123, 126
Tubal ligation, 131, 134
24-hour (Holter) ECG monitoring, 157

# U

Ultrasound, 160
Universal Sedation Form, 83–84
Urokinase, 158
Urologic surgery, 143–145

# V

Vaginal procedures, 132
Valium, 37, 39, 73
Vecuronium (Norcuron), 39
Versed, 37, 86, 118
Volume depletion, 168
Volume imbalance, 170

# W

"Wet tap," 53
Wisdom teeth, 141
Wound care, 111

# X

Xylocaine, 54, 95

# Z

Zantac, 170
Zofran, 99, 161
Zoladex, 161

# PRETEST ANSWER KEY

1. a Chapter 1
2. c Chapter 2
3. b Chapter 3
4. b Chapter 4
5. d Chapter 5
6. d Chapter 5
7. a Chapter 5
8. c Chapter 6
9. a Chapter 6
10. c Chapter 7
11. a Chapter 7
12. a Chapter 7
13. a Chapter 8
14. c Chapter 9
15. a Chapter 9
16. b Chapter 10
17. b Chapter 10
18. a Chapter 11
19. d Chapter 11
20. a Chapter 12
21. b Chapter 12
22. b Chapter 13
23. d Chatper 13
24. a Chapter 14
25. b Chapter 14

# NOTES

# NOTES

# NOTES

# NOTES